AGE
WELL
NOW

AGE WELL NOW

Body, Mind & Soul

S. Gottlieb and
F. Rosenberg-Gottlieb

Published 2021 by Gildan Media LLC
aka G&D Media
www.GandDmedia.com

Photograph of the authors (page 296) by Mendy Bleier

Front cover design by Tom McKeveny

Interior design by Meghan Day Healey of Story Horse, LLC.

Library of Congress Cataloging-in-Publication Data is available upon request

ISBN: 978-1-7225-0518-9

10 9 8 7 6 5 4 3 2 1

∾ ∾ ∾ ∾ ∾

*To the
children,
grandchildren,
adopted children,
stepchildren,
virtual children,
honorary children,
inner children,
former children,
and children-in-training
we are,
have been,
and will forever be.*

∾ ∾ ∾ ∾ ∾

Contents

Preface to the Second Edition

Since the original publication of the first edition, entitled *Awesome Aging*, we've been delighted by the responses of our readers. In workshops, book readings, and personal consultations throughout the U.S. and around the world, people of all ages and orientations have expressed their appreciation of the insights and guidance we have striven to convey. In many instances they have shared with us ongoing transformations in the quality of their lives.

We say, "of all ages," because the book's readership has extended far beyond our initial target audience of the over-fifty-five set. One friend asked why we didn't title the book *Awesome Living*, because he sees the book as relevant to every phase of our lives. After all, we've all been aging from the moment we left the womb. Just as it's never too late to reinvent oneself, so too is it never too early. The newfound freedom from jumping through hoops, so often characteristic of the third acts of our lives, can with a bit of imagination and determination be acquired during acts one and two as well.

In this second edition, we've therefore changed the title of the book—because one is never too young, and the moment is always ripe, to gain the wisdom and the grace of age—to *Age Well Now*.

Not long ago, we had the pleasure and privilege of appearing in a series of weekend speaking engagements at a beach community in Southern California. Among the attendees at our Saturday evening book reading was a sixty-something techie professional. In the Q&A session after our presentation, he told the crowd about the progress he felt he'd made in recent years through a men's group that met regularly in members' homes. He spoke about the personal goals he hadn't yet met. He then proceeded to complain, somewhat tongue in cheek, about the content of our talk. "Where was this information when we really needed it thirty years ago?"

It's often said these days that we live in interesting times—a catchphrase usually attributed to some ancient Chinese curse. Whether or not that's accurate, the irony is not lost on us in the twenty-first century. It means different things in different contexts, but one of the more poignant examples we've observed concerns the way the generations relate to one another. As life expectancies rise, young people have grown more convinced than ever that they've already mastered most of what there is to learn. In our naivete, we proudly address our principal readership as fellow baby boomers, only to discover that *boomer* has taken on a pejorative tone in popular culture. "OK Boomer," on Twitter and T-shirts, is now millennial-speak for "Sit down, shut up, and leave the driving to us."

We'll own that. Our generation is at least as responsible as our sons and daughters for the gradually waning evidence of mutual respect in today's fractious society. If youth refuses to defer to the wisdom of age, maybe it's because we seniors have modeled a similar attitude toward our elders. Or maybe the vaunted value of our accumulated life experience hasn't been bright enough, in and of itself, to shine them on. We could certainly be better examples, care more compassionately, demonstrate more integrity, and communicate more effectively.

That's been a major aspect of our intention in writing this book in the first place—to inspire, refine, and empower ourselves, not just to reinvent ourselves and enjoy our remaining decades, but also to represent the values and strengths we've acquired to the next generation. Our kids, grandkids, communities, and fellow humans are waiting for what we have to offer, whether or not they realize it yet.

There are, and probably always will be, moments when authors, artists, educators, or mentors recognize their own shortcomings. It can be painful to acknowledge one's own failure to fully and consistently embody the insights one wants to convey. The singer is rarely everything he or she purports to be in the song. We're no exception. We write, speak, and teach with great sincerity, for example, about loving and harmonious relationships, and yet occasionally find ourselves unequal to those ideals. (Occasionally? Perhaps more often than we'd like to admit.) In such situations, after being stymied and stuck for a while, we've sometimes turned to our own book to remind us of what we thought we knew, but clearly didn't know well enough.

Just last summer it happened: we were away from home, in the lovely mountains of upstate New York. For one of us it was a time of rest and recreation, and for the other it was a working vacation, with heavy emphasis on the working part. The dissonance was a bit too much to handle. Suddenly our interactions became far from harmonious; words flew, tempers flared. It wasn't very pretty. So we took a walk, sat together in a gazebo by the lake, and read to each other from the chapter entitled "Making Love Last." A few pages in, instead of the bickering, it was more like, "Oh, right! I knew we were forgetting something." And we laughed, and we returned to who we actually are. All better!

That sort of memory lapse is not an accident. Nor is it without purpose. Such incidents, together with numerous conversations we've had with readers during our book tour, have helped us add more meaning and practical significance to this book by tweaking the original text or adding a passage here or there. A new appendix concisely sums up seven useful, potentially life-changing habits. We've added a new chapter, sharing fresh new perspectives gained in the midst of global turmoil. And we've enhanced the chapter on health and wellness to include some insights into healing that go beyond our prior emphasis on preventive health habits. It adds further nuance to the idea of mindfulness, clarifying what it means to be fully present in the here and now, in the context of alleviating pain.

A human being is always a work in progress. So are the fruits of our labors. Please enjoy this new edition and continue to grow with us.

Simcha and Frumma Gottlieb
Miami, Florida
September 2020

Introduction
Better, Better, Better

Got to admit, it's getting better, a little better all the time.

—LENNON AND McCARTNEY

They called it the *baby boom*. Smack dab in the middle of the twentieth century, as the smoke from World War II was beginning to clear and very different kinds of battle lines were being drawn across the globe, a new generation popped up to say, "Hey! We're here. And you ain't seen nothing like us yet."

Right out of the womb, we were determined to be different. We cut our teeth on this amazing new toy called TV. We took full advantage of Dr. Spock's liberal prescription for permissive parenting. We saw unprecedented affluence emerging all around us, but were not all that impressed. Sinatra morphed into Elvis; street corner doo-wop became bigger than the big bands. As Neil Armstrong took his one small step on the moon, we were exploring uncharted territories of our own. By the time the Hubble telescope was sending back the first photographs of the outer reaches of the universe, we were embracing a more universal perspective than our great-grandparents could ever have imagined.

We were trendsetters, mold breakers. We didn't do adolescence, or college, or marriage, the way our elders had done. Some of us tuned in, turned on, and dropped out. Even those who dropped back in were more interested in fulfilling a personal vision than meeting others' expectations. Taking over Daddy's business was no longer the default option.

Filled with idealism, some of us started our careers in the Peace Corps or Vista, determined not just to see the world but to change it. Others (perhaps rebelling against the rebels) went to law school, medical school, or business school, leaving the revolution to the revolutionaries.

When it came time to start families, we reinvented natural childbirth with Lamaze classes and carried our babies in backpacks imported from Africa. We nurtured our souls with meditation from India, balanced our bodies with brown rice from Japan, pushed the envelope with grass from Panama, and made sense of it all with music from Liverpool. What had always been was not nearly as interesting to us as what we were able to envision but had not yet seen: the so-called reality in front of our faces wasn't far out enough. We grew disenchanted with conventional politics, embraced equality, scorned wars, and transformed social roles. We rejected the old-school paradigms we'd been spoon-fed, and reframed our cultural perspective in the bright new light of long-overlooked wisdom traditions. The world was our oyster. Even the sky was not the limit.

Act Three: Curtain Up

Now we're getting older. The first wave of baby boomers who came of age in the 1960s are well into *their* sixties now. The later arrivals, born in the 1960s, are now turning a corner and entering their sixth decade. The curtain is about to come up on what has been rather theatrically called the Third Act of our lives.

Are we where we thought we'd be? Perhaps, but more likely not. Career disappointments, financial setbacks, divorce, poor health—even the deaths of loved ones—one or more of these calamities has probably thrown us for a loop at some point. "Life is what happens," John Lennon famously sang, "when you're busy making other plans." He recorded that lyric at a turning point in his life—rising to a new beginning after having fallen into dark days from the heights of his career.

We've all made mistakes, been let down, let others down. Regrets are an inevitable part of the package and can dampen our enthusiasm—if we let them. Who among us hasn't experienced some measure of what's-the-point pessimism or been-there-done-that cynicism? We've been to the wars and back. We have allowed moments of failure or tragedy to harden into scars. But then there's that wizened wise person inside who recognizes that each of these mistakes can afford us insight and offer an opportunity to transform darkness into light.

We may at times think ourselves unfit because the muscle tone isn't what it once was or the skin has begun to sag. But that's a distortion, a reflection of an empty culture that puts more emphasis on the wrapping than on the gift within. Our most important muscles—mind and heart—are stronger than they've ever been, because for decades we've been bench-pressing the heavy loads of life. The part of us that can never be diminished is our spirit. It is boundless, infinite; it remains pure and powerful and shines on nonstop even as we slog through the mud and muck.

That indomitable spirit is both our inspiration and our engine. It imbues us with the will to put it to work. And we've seen it working. We know octogenarians who are succeeding in brand-new second and third careers, grandmas who run marathons, geezers who have discarded old expectations to become entrepreneurs, mastering technologies of which they had never before dared to dream. We too have dared to dream, and you can too.

We are committed to aging well. We are determined to perform Act Three with style and grace, staying mindful and joyful and focused and fit. We will rewrite our scripts when necessary to redeem the lapses, failings, and unfinished business left over from Acts One and Two. After all these years—after all the laughter and the tears, the trial and error, the wins and losses and lessons learned—nothing can stop us from getting our act together and living lives that meet and exceed our own highest aspirations.

This, then, is our intention with this book: to help ensure that we all make our Third Acts spectacular. It is about the ways we think and feel and speak and behave; the values that drive our lives, the purpose we pursue, the habits we develop, and the fabrics we use to weave our tapestries. We may not always be able to choose the situations or control the people in our lives, but we can always choose the way we respond.

There will undoubtedly be more troubles ahead: losses, disappointments, illnesses—obstacles that challenge our energy and optimism. But with the problems comes freedom—freedom to choose perspective, cultivate consciousness, and live with integrity and equanimity. If we live in harmony with our innermost values, we can reclaim and reimagine the vision of our youth. If we will embrace our passion with unbridled enthusiasm, we might just realize the promise of that old sixties certainty that we are *getting better all the time.*

A Brief Word about the Authors

The coauthors, Simcha and Frumma, have each worn a wide variety of hats in the course of their collective 120-plus years. The former is the child of a self-described anarchist revolutionary from the East Village; the latter was raised by a Park Avenue Republican stockbroker.

While Frumma was serving in the domestic Peace Corps on the island of Kauai, Simcha was touring America with an avant-garde theatrical troupe. As the 1960s were winding down, Simcha found himself owning and operating one of the East Coast's first natural foods restaurants, under the tutelage of one of that movement's leading healers, Michel Abehsera (whose books Simcha later edited).

Frumma was co-founder of an innovative chain of successful health food stores in Colorado that later evolved (after Frumma had moved on to other, less lucrative pursuits) into a couple of corporate giants that have become household names today. Do the names Celestial Seasonings and Whole Foods ring a bell?

We both became educators along the way, from early childhood programs through graduate school lecture halls; in adult education workshops, meditation tutorials, and online seminars. Frumma became the principal of a large, highly regarded private day school, as well as a beloved teacher, an internationally respected educational consultant, and a much sought-after life coach. Simcha administered a groundbreaking fellowship program for elite college students and—after returning to graduate school himself to become a clinical practitioner of herbal medicine and acupuncture—was a professor of Chinese medicine.

Where We're Coming From

The thread that runs through all these diverse pursuits is a fascination with the technology, so to speak, of personal change. Over the years, in our various lectures, articles, coaching, and clinical relationships, we've often focused on *emotional intelligence*. Intellectual insights may be nifty, but if we fail to feel the feelings, how on earth will we walk the walk?

The literature of psychology and self-help is well stocked with assiduously researched guidelines in the art of aligning the head and heart. Some methods are helpful

THE BLUE ZONE

What do Okinawa, Japan, Nicoya, Greece, and Loma Linda, California, have in common? They are communities around the world identified as having the highest concentration of centenarians. Scientists call them Blue Zones; research has pinpointed the lifestyle choices that help people live long, robust lives to the age of one hundred and beyond:

- *Active engagement in family and social life*
- *A clearly defined sense of life purpose*
- *Regular exercise and other methods of stress reduction*
- *Moderate caloric intake and a primarily plant-based diet*
- *Engagement in meaningful spiritual or religious pursuits*

This zone, of course, is not limited to any particular locale. It's an internalized way of life. Read on, and explore with us such life-supporting principles and more—a full spectrum of practices and attitudes, and the ideas that lie behind them. Longevity entails more than mere numbers of years; it is about quality of life.

for some of us, and others for others. Relevance and efficacy are largely a function of personal resonance. There is no one-size-fits-all.

We have found, moreover, that *getting better all the time* calls for not just the integration of intellect and emotion, but well-being in all four dimensions of life: physical, emotional, cognitive, and spiritual.

As you will see, our approach is toward the cultivation of whole health—from our physical bodies and behavior to the innermost sensibilities of the soul. We want you to feel good all over, inside and out, and in a sustained and ever more meaningful way. We evaluate these methods and perspectives not just for pragmatic efficacy, but also in the context of a whole-systems worldview—an ecology of self-development, so that no part of us is cultivated at the expense of another part. That's the way to stay whole and make love last.

Our spiritual sources and the wisdom traditions from which we draw sustenance have evolved over the years, from eclectic, exploratory, and multicultural to an in-depth devotion to the specific cultural legacy of our Hebrew ancestry. While some of our past writings and lectures have been addressed primarily to co-religionists and are based on scriptural, rabbinical, or kabbalistic teachings, we are focused here on universally applicable wisdom that is accessible to everyone and useful to all.

This is a nondenominational, nonsectarian book. Although it is unabashedly faith-based at its core, we've intentionally kept its language and its context secular. We expect you'll find good guidance here even if your own belief system and cultural frame of reference differ from ours.

When friends hear us say that we write together, they often ask what sort of process and/or pitfalls that entails. Interesting question. How in fact do two people with deeply entrenched, markedly different sensibilities, opinions, and work habits manage to speak with one voice?

Especially husband and wife? The short smart-aleck answer might be "with great difficulty." But our hope is that some longer and more meaningful answers will become apparent in the course of this book. You will find, however, that from time to time we've each found it appropriate to pipe up as individuals, with a personal anecdote or divergent point of view. These passages will appear from time to time as sidebars. We've resisted the temptation to color-code them pink and blue.

Navigating this Book

This book is structured in three parts. Part One is about setting our intentions—outlining the themes of our Third Act. Part Two delves more deeply into the development of character—the inner work that renders us heroes rather than bit players. And Part Three goes into greater detail, fleshing out specific scenarios as they unfold in our relationships, in all the compartments of our lives. (Not that our lives are actually compartmentalized—it's all one seamless story!)

You will probably benefit most from reading these chapters sequentially. However, if you're like us and tend to sneak to the back of a book or poke around randomly before making a commitment, feel free. Any given chapter can also stand alone, and will probably lead you back to the beginning anyway. The best way to read this book is the way you choose.

Note also that a few specific practical exercises will appear from time to time as sidebars for easy reference.

It also bears mentioning that, although we are primarily addressing our Third Act, baby boomer peers, the reader needn't be "of a certain age" to appreciate and gain from this book. Sagacity is not restricted to us elders. Some of our closest and cleverest friends are of more tender years.

Coming Unstuck

To genuinely and authentically feel *younger than yesterday* calls for a shift in our attitude toward time. We're not alone in noting that negative emotion is often bound up with being somehow stuck in time or unable to go with the flow. We are often anxious about the future, remorseful about the past. The history of our past mistakes and old bad habits can weigh us down like the proverbial ball and chain; our hopes for the future can sometimes generate the opposite of hope—pessimism, resistance, or fear.

We can learn how to rise above anxiety and regret. Astute guides of both ancient and modern vintage have pointed out the extraordinary benefits of being simply present in the moment, in the here and now—surfing, so to speak, on the crest of the wave of time. And mystics of many persuasions have taught us how this ability to "be here now" paradoxically connects us with an eternal, timeless dimension of reality. We can become neither young nor old, neither naive nor jaded, as alive and unburdened and invincible as a child running from Adventureland to Fantasyland to Tomorrowland with nary a care.

On the other hand, let's face it: the clock is ticking. We have a history; the future looms. But not in a bad way, if we can figure out how to sustain that sense of timeless spontaneity while doing all the grownup things we've been trained to do, like remembering our responsibilities and planning for those inevitable dark and stormy nights. Most of us were under a fair amount of pressure during our First and Second Acts, while raising families, building careers, paying dues and bills, and fighting battles we may or may not have chosen. Harrowing at times, was it not? Well, take a deep breath and consider: how does it feel now? Do we continue to react to that sense of pressure *even when it's no longer there?*

We're not suggesting that there aren't challenges. There are, and they're sometimes serious. The golden opportunity now, however, is to marshal the hard-won wisdom we've acquired on the battlefields and put it to work.

Through many days and decades tethered to our clocks, calendars, and computers, we've discovered a thing or two about how to be here now with joy and peace of mind. There's plenty more to learn and therefore to share— because sharing is the best way to keep learning. Together we can continue to patch up the holes in our histories, glee-fully meet our destinies, and put one sure foot in front of the other along this still long, still winding road.

The beginning is embedded in the end,
and the end in the beginning.

—SEFER YETZIRAH

PART ONE

If life is a journey, its true significance is found
not only in its starting point and destination but in
the inner experience of each step along the way.

Where we are is truly meaningful only in light of *who* we are.

Before embarking, let us free ourselves from the
roadblocks and wrong turns that impede our progress,
from the internal maze that can lead us astray.

To chart our itinerary, we begin with introspection:

"What are my true desires, my joys and fears? What dreams,
commitments, and goals define my life? Is my mission aligned
with my desire? Do my actions embody my intent?

"Am I over the hill, or shall I still keep climbing?"

1

Me Tarzan!

*The two most important days in your life are the day
you are born and the day you find out why.*

—MARK TWAIN

Once upon a simpler time, age signified wisdom. Traditional societies saw their elders as sages, models of emotional stability and equanimity, reliable sources of sound advice acquired through rich life experience.

Our present-day ageist culture has supplanted that badge of honor with ridicule. The modern image of senior citizens is one of doddering ditzes or grumpy old men who can barely get through an early-bird special without nodding off, and then forgetting where they parked the car. Until very recently, even the medical literature tended to reinforce this mythology with theories of cognitive decline.

But today we're finding that the more rigorous and penetrating science supports a more upbeat scenario for seniors.

As the average life expectancy rises and positive psychology gains currency, it's becoming more difficult to deny that we're on the way *up*. The arcs of our life stories need not end in a downward slope.

Perhaps Jane Fonda (looking fabulous, by the way, in her eighth decade) said it most cogently in her recent TED Talks presentation:

> I have come to find that a more appropriate metaphor for aging is a staircase—the upward ascension of the human spirit, bringing us into wisdom, wholeness and authenticity. Age not at all as pathology; age as potential. . . . Most people over fifty feel better, are less stressed, are less hostile, less anxious. . . . Some of the studies even say we're happier.[1]

New neurological research reveals that while younger people may have better short-term memory and absorb new bits of information more readily, older people are more adept at connecting the dots: associative thinking, complex reasoning, seeing the big picture. According to Dr. Gary Small, professor of psychiatry and Director of the UCLA Longevity Center, "The older brain is quite resilient and can be stimulated to innovate, create and contribute in extraordinary ways."[2]

Well, then, what shall we create? How shall we leverage our abundance of life experience and enhanced capacity for rescuing the universe from ruin?

Take a moment to consider this conversation in *Alice's Adventures in Wonderland* between Alice and the Cheshire Cat:

> "Would you please tell me which way I ought to walk from here?"
>
> "That depends a good deal on where you want to get to," said the Cat.
>
> "I don't much care where," said Alice.
>
> "Then it doesn't matter which way you walk."[3]

It matters. We care. To get a good start, we need a clear idea of where we are going and why. To put all the potential wisdom of our seasoned, mature minds to work, we need to refine and define the vision. The Cheshire Cat won't do that for us.

On a Clear Day You Can See Forever

It's entirely possible that you may have lived through five decades or more without ever having composed a personal mission statement. In fact, most of us haven't. How many of us have had the time, the patience, and the sense of freedom to make a clearly articulated, well-conceived declaration of why we are here and what we want to accomplish in life? From our earliest beginnings, we've been busy meeting the expectations of others, fulfilling responsibilities that were thrust upon us, or pursuing goals that seemed like a good idea at the time.

The lucky ones got it right and chose a craft, a career, or a calling they enjoyed and at which they could succeed—and they succeeded. Some achieved job satisfaction, financial success, or honor, but at the expense of an unfulfilled dream or a nagging sense of "something missing." Some had more than one career, reinventing themselves for fun and profit, chasing rainbows or pots of gold. Others found more frustration than fulfillment.

Even if it all works out well, there comes a time in life when you turn a corner and say, "What now?"

The First Act of every life story is about setting the stage, developing character, establishing the challenge. The Second Act is where the plot thickens and the action, the drama, the comedy and romance begin to play hot and heavy. The third act—ah! The *Third Act*! This is when things start to get really interesting. This is where the true purpose of a life can come to light.

Childhood was a time when we were surprised at every turn, finding fun in every mud puddle or pile of leaves. As our long stories have unfolded, as we've grappled with life's vicissitudes, we've lost that sense of wonder and surprise. Or at least we think we have. Truth is, we've still got it. It's just that now we have to dig a little deeper and remember how to surprise *ourselves*.

Perhaps you've never really had a well-defined sense of your life's purpose—you were too busy jumping through hoops. Or maybe you did, but is it working for you now? Does it still ring true? Now may be the time to reexamine old assumptions and write—or rewrite—your mission

CHEKHOV'S GUN

The famous Russian playwright Anton Chekhov, discussing the finer points of his craft, once remarked that if you place a pistol or rifle on the wall in the first act of your drama, you'd better be sure that it is fired in the third act.

It works that way in reverse as well. As we enter the Third Act of our lives, we're working on the rewrite. One of the ways to guarantee an exciting and satisfying finale is to look back into our first and second acts. What dreams, desires, unfinished business, or unfulfilled intentions are yet to be resolved? Was there some "gun" hanging on one of our walls that hasn't yet been fired? It might just turn out to be the key to our happy ending.

statement. Good news: now you have the time to do it. It's a perk of a certain age.

Perhaps you don't agree? Maybe you still feel that you're too busy, too distracted, or too tired to find out who you want to be when you *really* grow up? In our modern, complex technological world, we can easily lose touch, and not just with our environment. We can actually forget who we are.

It wasn't like that in simpler times. Take the classic story of *Tarzan the Ape Man* by Edgar Rice Burroughs, first published in 1912.[4] Abandoned in the jungle as a tiny child, he grew up without having to deal with the expectations of overbearing parents. He didn't need to cope with agenda-driven school curricula or standardized testing that all but obliterated his own inclinations and sensibilities. He didn't have to submit to performance assessment or peer review. From his very first bit of dialogue, he makes it perfectly clear that he knows exactly who he is, and precisely what he wants:

"Me Tarzan. You Jane."

Though he may be a fictional character, Tarzan is a great role model. He represents the quintessence of what it means to be free. Not that he has no roles to play or purpose to pursue. He'll gladly leap into action to protect the pristine beauty of the jungle from greedy, thieving, ivory hunters, or to save Jane from a hungry crocodile. But he doesn't need to attend a webinar or hire a life coach to live a life of authenticity. He simply beats his chest in unabashed joy and swings freely from tree to tree.

Freedom means a lot of things to different people in different contexts. Circumstances may present us with limitations, real or imagined. But we've found that there's one universal sign of being truly free, regardless of situational constraints: the ability to choose what you will do with your time. If you want that freedom, if you want to get in touch with your inner Tarzan, you can.

We'll be speaking in later chapters about time management, time wasters, and something we call *time affluence* (see chapter 3). We'll even touch upon a kind of time travel. But for now let's seize the moment and cut to the chase. In these opening moments of Act Three the task at hand is to focus on recognizing your true sense of purpose in life. It's time to get down to the core, to the real nitty-gritty.

For most of us, by the time we were knee deep into the Second Act of our lives, we had little wiggle room. As businesspeople or professionals, tradesmen or craftsmen, creative types or entrepreneurs, whatever the colors of our collars or the size of our families, our days were well-defined. We assumed roles, took on responsibilities, ticked off items on to-do lists, paid bills and tuitions and dues. This kind of intensely organized or programmed lifestyle has certain advantages. In fact, research has shown that our minds become more comfortable with predictable patterns. We are more at ease when we have a clear sense of schedule. We may even identify such a tightly planned way of life as what it means to be an adult.

But our patterns change as we mature. There's a continuing shift in the quality of our lives as time goes by. To be in flow, we need to recognize the changes and adjust accordingly. (For more details on what it means to be in flow, see chapter 4.) For example, as the kids grow up and leave home, we experience a different sense of urgency. We gain more discretionary time and can afford to become more selective and introspective about how we spend that time. But if we don't immediately perceive that shift, we may persist in feeling a sense of emergency when there is none, or of emptiness in the absence of external demands.

Because we don't know what is really important to us, everything seems important.

The same is true in our jobs. Many of us work fewer hours (at least on paper) than when our careers were climbing toward their peak. If we are able to acknowledge and embrace that reality, time becomes more elective, and our options expand. But we may not yet be relaxed enough to notice. This can be rougher for some of us than for others. If we were employees and our schedules were handed to us, the ability to freely choose what we will do with our time calls for a new set of skills.

Then there are those of us who have joined, or are about to join, the ten thousand baby boomers a day who are defined as "retired." So you used to be a doctor, a lawyer, a plumber, a construction worker, a teacher, or a CPA? What are you now? Archived? Mothballed? No longer functional? In our humble opinion, what a waste of talent! Why not reframe "retired" into "redefined"?

Having reinvented ourselves numerous times during our twelve-plus collective decades on this planet, the two of us have explored many different methods of sorting priorities and clarifying a sense of purpose. Some were gleaned from such seminal guides as *How to Get Control of Your Time and Your Life* and *What Color is Your Parachute?* (first published in the 1970s) and the still best-selling, still relevant, Stephen Covey classic *Seven Habits of Highly Effective People*. Through the ensuing years of experience as both clients and coaches, we also gained terrific insight into the myriad devious devices we all employ in order to stay stuck. Of necessity, we continued to deepen our perspective with an eclectic array of studies in psychology, neuroscience, medicine, emotional intelligence, meditation, biophysics, and philosophy. Most significantly, we have evaluated these methods and their philosophical foundations in the light of profound wisdom traditions that have, from time immemorial, provided tried-and-true roadmaps to what Thomas Jefferson enshrined as the "pursuit of happiness." (Yes, "life" and "liberty" come with the territory too.)

All that said and done, we humbly recommend at this point that you begin your journey toward your inner Tarzan with an exercise that is very simple. The process begins by delving into and gaining awareness of your deepest abiding sense of what matters to you most—what Stephen Covey calls your "governing values." Everything else will follow from there (though not necessarily automatically . . . stay tuned.)

EVALUATING VALUES

Covey, among other expert coaches, encourages people to refine their focus by creating a list of the core concepts that mean the most to them personally, inwardly. These are the values that motivate us, that drive our behavior and ultimately determine our most powerful decisions. It's important to identify the values that are genuinely meaningful to you as an individual, regardless of others' concerns or expectations. Have a look at the sample list on the next page and consider which among them may resonate for you.

SOME MEANINGFUL VALUES

Honesty	*Tranquility*	*Courage*
Family	*Beauty*	*Security*
Creativity	*Respect*	*Equanimity*
Spirituality	*Gratitude*	*Community*
Kindness	*Faith*	*Humor*
Service	*Freedom*	*Responsibility*
Industry	*Loyalty*	*Integrity*
Justice	*Generosity*	*Charity*
Wealth	*Patience*	*Teamwork*
Health	*Trust*	*Fitness*
Orderliness	*Compassion*	*Leadership*
Cleanliness	*Quality*	*Wisdom*

Though all these values are worthy, we encourage you to compose a list of the governing values in *your* life. Think about what is most meaningful and motivating *to you*—not because you've been told or taught that it's a good idea, but because it's consistent with *who you are.* You'll soon see how identifying these values can make the difference between a satisfying, successful Third Act and a life of frustration and regret. These principles will drive your choices; they are the engine that will take you where you want to go, the foundation upon which you will create your personal mission statement.

Allow us to guide you through this exercise. It's outlined for easy reference in the accompanying sidebar. It shouldn't take more than a half hour or so to go through all the steps; any more than that, and you may be over-thinking the task.

These questions often come up at this stage of the game: How do I know if a value is consistent with who I am? Am I my thoughts? My feelings? What if I think it's a good idea to be, for example, generous, but when push comes to shove, I tend to be more like a Scrooge? Maybe I really *am* a cheap, stingy son-of-a-whatever!

Or perhaps you really want to say you believe in team-work, but for most of your life effective collaboration has

EXERCISE ONE: GOVERNING VALUES

On a blank, unlined sheet of paper (yes, paper; do this by hand, not on a keyboard, so that it comes more directly from the heart) write down your personal list of the fifteen or twenty values that mean the most to you, one word to a line. Take your time.

Go over the list, open your inner intuitive eye, and con-sider your priorities. Think about which items are more important and which are less significant; assign a number to each from 1 to 5: 1 for those that are indispensable, 5 for the ones you think you could live without.

Take a new page and write down the values to which you assigned the numbers 1 or 2. If there are more than five, pri-oritize again. Pare down the list until you have no more than five items, and no fewer than three. These are your govern-ing values. We'll be basing your next steps on this list. Don't worry if you're a little uncertain about it. There will be ample opportunity to revisit the vision as we proceed.

been difficult to achieve. In fact, your best work has been accomplished on your own, the hard way. So which is your true value—*teamwork* or rugged individualism? How can we discern our governing values if our minds, our hearts, and our experiences in the trenches don't align?

CONGRUENCE

Psychologist Carl Rogers and his followers called this alignment *congruence*. It means that the person you would ideally *like to be* is consistent with the way you *actually behave*, that the story you tell yourself is more or less the same as the face you present to the world. We prefer to refer to it more simply as being whole or uncomplicated— or at least (because human beings *are* complex) being capable of resolving inner conflicts when they inevitably arise. Such wholeness empowers us to become amazingly greater than merely the sum of our parts. We'll have more to say throughout the book about getting all our parts aligned.

After redefining your core values, it can be challenging to integrate them seamlessly with old, entrenched feelings and habits. You may well find it necessary to revisit Exercise One later in light of the insights you'll discover in upcoming chapters. In fact, it can be worthwhile to reexamine your core values from time to time, either independently or in the workshops we offer (see our contact information at the back of this book.)

But for now, don't worry about perfection. Let's take a shot at identifying the *ideal* you, and the *real* you will catch up soon enough.

When you have identified your values, take a moment to bring them to life. Use your imagination to evoke a mental picture and an emotional sense of what it will look like and feel like when you are living that value.

For example, say one of your core values is *service*. Play with it: "When I am living the value of *service*, I set aside time each week to serve people who are less fortunate. I volunteer for the Friendship Circle and the Food Bank, giving each organization two hours of my time per week. The smiling faces nourish me . . ."

Or *tranquility*: "I meditate or pray for twenty minutes twice daily. I remind myself that nothing happens by accident, that the tests I face are for my benefit. In fact they may well serve to enhance my personal growth, and I welcome them. It feels like my life is unfolding exactly as it should."

When you express these visualizations in the present tense, they become more palpable rather than merely something you might do when you have time someday. Envisioning yourself living your value renders it more likely that you will make choices that align with your priorities. You will better recognize the difference between what seems urgent (that is, motivated by stress) and what is truly important (value-driven.) You become empowered to make better choices in planning the week, or in the moment.

So that's our first exercise—a powerful place to start. A wholesome, satisfying life begins not with empty hedonism, but with the specific joy that comes only from a life lived with meaning and purpose. Your values provide your cornerstone.

HAVING DIFFICULTY?

You may be experiencing a bit of resistance to going through this exercise just about now. Maybe you're all about spontaneity, or perhaps you think these techniques are a waste of time. We understand. Between the two of us, Simcha is more susceptible to such reluctance, whereas Frumma thrives on this sort of activity.

In situations like this, Stephen Covey deploys a parable about a woodchopper who thinks he has no time to sharpen his ax. He spends all day splitting logs that would have been chopped in an hour if he'd taken ten minutes to sharpen the blade.

Here's a slightly more apt parable. Let's say you're in an early phase of life—call it Act Two—and seeking to create your dream career. If you don't take a little time to formulate a vision of what that looks like, you'll never know what you want—and you'll end up working for someone who does.

Now consider the same scenario as it applies to Act Three: without that vision, things may end up not working very well at all.

When we first began to write this book, we came up against an enormous amount of inertia that kept us from gaining the momentum we needed to get it done. It became almost embarrassing to be repeatedly described as the "authors of the forthcoming book" while the keyboards of our computers gathered dust for the better part of two years. One night we were supposed to attend an engagement party of a close friend. It seemed important; it was certainly urgent. But something told us that if we stayed home that night because we are *writers*, we might just come unstuck. At that moment, we made a pivotal decision.

But we weren't entirely there yet. Some old attitudes and habits still stood in our way. Read on as we explore the next phase of transforming meaningful values into real life.

Tarzan makes it look easy. His most extraordinary skill is his ability to let go of the vine he's holding on to so that he can complete the leap and grab hold of the next one. Having taken the first step of envisioning the trees we want to swing in, we now need to master the art of releasing the vine we've been dangling from. Turn the page: the next vine is just ahead.

❧ 2 ❧

Passions, Roles, and Goals

The only person you are destined to
become is the person you decide to be.
—RALPH WALDO EMERSON

There are two kinds of hypocrites. A dishonest hypocrite tries to fool the world and get away with it. There's not much we have to say to these folks, other than "Sooner or later you'll figure out that what goes around comes around." Honest hypocrites, on the other hand, have nobler intentions; they just set standards for themselves that they can't consistently fulfill.

As heartfelt as our ideal values may seem to be, when push comes to shove we may find ourselves coming up short in the strength-of-character department. "I *meant* to have a strong work ethic." "Altruism seemed like a good idea at the time." "My commitments were ironclad when I made them, but . . ." And we rationalize, and excuse ourselves: "Nobody's perfect." "The heart wants what it wants." "Nice guys finish last." "Look how many people have less integrity than I do." "After all, sometimes in this nasty world, the mature response is compromise." So it happens that the good ship *Core Values* crashes on the rocky shores of reality.

Having defined ourselves conceptually in terms of our cherished values, what happens when the heart boogies to the beat of a somewhat different drum?

As baby boomers, many of us have been juggling mixed messages most of our lives. We've bought the line that we must do what we love—"follow your bliss!" Yet the demands of responsibility often render such advice impractical. There's frequently a disconnect between the governing values we embrace in our more sober moments and the passions that light our fires.

. . . .

SIMCHA'S SHRINK

In my early thirties, I spent a year or so in psychotherapy. As I bared my soul, the good doc would often interrupt and ask, "How do you feel about that?" I'd proceed to regale him with my explanations, theories, and rationales; whereupon, he'd repeat, "No, how do you feel about that?"

It took me a while to figure out that what I thought were feelings were often not feelings at all. I was merely thinking about feelings, all up in my head, imagining I was in touch with my heart. Intellect has a way of masquerading as emotion, and vice versa. This problem, however, is its own solution: it points to the fact that intellect and emotion include each other.

. . . .

No mission statement will be complete or true if it addresses only our conceptual best values and fails to embody our passionate desires. Values alone, though central to defining our life's purpose, can be impotent. Passion gets us going, keeps us moving, and gets it done. So we're going to pay some attention in this chapter to identifying our passion(s) in life. First, however, let's have a glance at where passions lie on the map of human experience.

Tug-of-War: Between Heart and Head

Sadly—at times tragically—human beings experience conflict between the cool, collected conclusions of the discerning mind and the blazing passions of the heart. The struggle between intellect and emotion can make for some pretty gripping psychological drama.

But it isn't necessarily always so. Other ways of managing this dynamic relationship can help us transform antagonism into collaboration, enmity into interdependence.

At the risk of oversimplifying: the brain is the seat of reason, and the heart the home of our emotions—love and fear, attraction and aversion, kindness and constraint. Neither the brain nor the heart is an island unto itself; they feed each other and form each other. For example, we would not *love* something or someone if we did not *understand* and *know* it, him, or her to be lovable. In this sense, the heart is by nature secondary to the mind; our emotions emerge as a result of a well-developed cognitive process. This has been described by some as the healthiest relationship between mind and heart, with the rational mind in charge, while the emotions remain subservient, under control. Theoretically, according to this point of view, all we need is the correct information, and we'll surely love what's worth loving and avoid what's not.

Alas, it doesn't always work that way. Sometimes the heart just won't comply. And maybe that's not as negative as it appears to the rationalist or the control freak. Particularly in these more emotionally liberated times, it's become fashionable to see the heart as nobler, purer, more authentic, and less devious than the mind. There's some merit to this point of view. History's greatest poets, composers, and visual artists would certainly concur.

It's a way of life, however, that more often than not spells trouble. Unruly emotion can back up on the brain like acid reflux after a greasy meal. Desire—sweet, seductive desire—or its opposite, a fear, a phobia, an allergic reaction, can hijack our most cherished values and corrupt our highest ideals. Unbridled passion, ego, and ambition can make mincemeat of reason. We'll spare you the sordid details of what this might look like in real life. Chances are you've seen what we mean.

But wait a second—what then do we do with "follow your bliss"? Is it not the heart's passionate desire for good that drives human creativity, productivity, achievement? Do what you love, we are told, and success will surely follow.

Humankind does not live by passion alone. Love may make the birds sing and the flowers grow and the planets spin; but we are neither animal, vegetable, nor mineral. We are *Homo sapiens*, and *sapiens* is the Latin word for *discerning*. A mind is a terrible thing to underrate.

So the revised model of a truly successful, fully realized, well-balanced, *whole* human being must embody passion, reason, and governing values singing in three-part harmony. It's a two-way street on a three-dimensional landscape. Neither the mind nor the heart nor any other part seeks to dominate; they nourish one another—generously, symbiotically, selflessly.

At this point you may well be thinking, "Yeah, right." OK, we agree, it's not so simple. But it's doable if we know how to navigate the terrain. We will soon revisit this map of human motivation and intention and develop a more fully fleshed-out model of who we are and how we roll.

EXERCISE TWO: IDENTIFYING YOUR PASSION(S)

Having gotten a bead on our core values in the previous chapter, the next step in the crystallization of our mission statements is an exercise that's a bit more, well, touchy-feely. Call it a checkup from the neck down.

This is the Passion Test, and it's pretty simple. In fact if you don't find it simple, it's not a true Passion Test. (We are indebted for this material to Chris and Janet Atwood. More details can be found in their book, appropriately titled *The Passion Test*.)[5]

Children, like Tarzan, do not need an exercise to analyze themselves and discover what they really love. They just do whatever they're doing until it's not fun anymore, and then they stop. We, however, who have been in the work force or in positions of responsibility for seemingly endless decades, may have had the spontaneity drilled out of us. We'll have to train ourselves to vacate all those musts, shoulds, ought to's, and got to's. Simplicity doesn't come easy.

PASSION TEST, STEP 1:

Sit in a quiet spot with a pad and pencil (or a laptop or tablet if you must) and take a few minutes to breathe and release. Close your eyes, and open your mind and heart. If you have a specific meditation practice, settle in with that for a moment or so. (If you don't, no worries; we'll be offering some suggestions later for your consideration.)

Open your eyes, and write: "When my life is ideal, when I am exactly where I want to be, with whom I want to be, and doing what I love to do, I am . . ."

Be courageous and honest. Drop the inhibitions and doubts. Do not concern yourself with whether it's possible or likely, or whether people will think you're nuts. Write at least ten different passions, ten juicy scenarios. A few examples:

I am . . .

. . . sitting in a chaise longue on a tropical beach, writing my third best seller.

. . . surrounded by grandchildren, telling them stories from the family lore.

. . . meditating daily and basking in inner peace.

. . . climbing Mount Everest, uploading my photos to *National Geographic*.

. . . belting out a song in a karaoke bar, drunk out of my mind.

Feel these fantasies. Don't give your inner critic a voice, and don't worry about the "hows"—just get the "whats" down. What are you doing? Where are you? What does it look like through your eyes? What do you feel?

Now let it rest a while. Sleep on it. Give your initial impulses a chance to ripen into sustainable emotions. Come back to them tomorrow with a fresh perspective, and work on the Passion Test, step 2.

PASSION TEST, STEP 2:

Compare your entries one to another to determine which among them are really the closest to your true desire.

If you could have either 1 or 2, which one would you choose? Then do the same between 3 and 4. Then take those two choices and compare them with 5. Which two would you prefer if you could only have two out of three?

And so on. Move on to the next set of choices, and then compare those selections with your previous selections. Don't worry if it feels as if you are giving up something important to you; just note that feeling and allow yourself to reconsider the choice that left you feeling that way.

For example, after examining the five passions cited above, you may decide that your best seller and your grandchildren are closer to your heart than the rest. Write those down, and don't be afraid to let go of the others.

If some of the comparisons lead to internal conflict, ask yourself, "Which of these alternatives would make me feel more fulfilled, more content with myself, more personally enriched?" There's no pressure here and no wrong answer; in real life you can have both choices, maybe even all—why not? The intention of this exercise is to arrive at some emotional clarity, not necessarily to make firm decisions.

Be honest with yourself, and try not to be influenced by what others might think. Many discover that their initial impulse is the truest. Keep going until you have identified your top five passions.

That's it. Set this exercise aside and absorb it from a distance. We'll return soon to your results. So far we've honed in on governing *values*, and heartfelt *passions*. With that in hand, let's now move on to consider two more down-to-earth aspects of what our lives are about, as we further clarify our mission in life, our sense of purpose, the *raison d'être* of our Third Act: *roles* and *goals*.

Roles and Goals

Many of us find ourselves juggling personae like circus performers spinning plates in the air. Our various, often incongruous roles are defined by our professions, avocations, and recreations; by our family ties, community connections, societal expectations, and secret ruminations. At times the roles can conflict, not just in terms of scheduling our finite, twenty-four-hour days and seven-day weeks, but even in a single moment. At this moment, right now, am I a teacher, a student, a parent, a spouse? A mentor, a disciple, a grandparent, a friend?

From a broader and deeper perspective, to what extent should I see myself as an individual with unique gifts and dreams? To what extent must I temper my individuality in accordance with duties and loyalties to the groups to which I belong?

As a life coach, Frumma is often called upon to guide a client in defining, prioritizing, and attending to multiple roles. In which roles are we doing well? Which need massaging? Which leave us with a nagging feeling that we've been guilty of neglect? This can be an important facet of harmonizing an otherwise chaotic lifestyle. Though a full treatment of how we go about it is beyond the scope of this book, one rule of thumb we'll share here is that it's important to do *something* in service of each of our roles *every week*. We can put these activities on our calendars in the same nonnegotiable way we schedule our dentist appointments.

Another suggestion (this one might be more difficult): while you are playing a particular role, whichever one it may be, be *all about* that role. Don't agonize inwardly over office politics while ostensibly listening to your spouse . . . and so forth, with respect to all activities. Do one thing, and only one thing, at a time. To be *100 percent present* in the task at hand is challenging. It's also the secret to success. Multitasking might be an enviable skill in some contexts, but it often lowers the quality of your life.

A key aspect of defining *yourself* is understanding who you are and what your intention is in different *contexts*. You are not your roles; but to be truly yourself, and true *to* yourself, it's important to be clear about your roles and how you apply yourself to them.

EXERCISE THREE: ROLE CALL

This exercise is straightforward enough: write down a list of your roles in life. Try to limit the number to seven. By way of illustration, here's a recent list Frumma drew up for herself:

> *I am: a wife, a mother, a grandmother, a spiritual mentor, an inspirational speaker, a writer, a coach, and a realtor.*

Oops—that's eight. Our suggestion that you shoot for no more than seven roles is carefully considered; on the other hand, it is a bit arbitrary. Maybe you can be a little more flexible on the number. Or, as Frumma continues:

> *Maybe I ought to drop one. I remember in elementary school having to draw a circle around the picture of the object that doesn't belong. At first glance, that looks like "realtor"—it's not nearly as aligned with my passion as the others.*
>
> *But the truth is I need the cash flow to enable those other roles. Not everything I do needs to feed my passion—some roles can just feed my face!*

Wait a minute . . . Aha! If I call myself a wise and loving matriarch, I can compress mother and grandmother into one.

- -

Wife	*Inspirational speaker*
~~*Mother*~~	
~~*Grandmother*~~	*Writer*
^*Matriarch*	*Coach*
Spiritual mentor	*Realtor*

- -

Just don't try that with your "spouse" role. That's a role that can't be compressed. In a sense, it's the one relationship that serves most effectively as a crucible for personal transformation. For those of us who are so blessed, marriage provides an accessible healing environment—a context in which we can most readily reclaim our wholeness. There will be more about this in chapter 9, as well as more about how to make that happen if you are not currently fortunate enough to be in the happiest of relationships.

INNER DESIRE STEPS OUT

At this point we can expand our model of how mind and heart interact and gain further insight into how our inner being—as defined by core values and passions—interfaces with our roles in the external world.

Whether we are artists or laborers, professionals or executives, parents or partners or all of the above, our roles are our arms of outreach. Although all these commitments, responsibilities, and relationships are important to us, they do not define us. Having acquired a deeper, more focused awareness of the *values* and *passions* that comprise your inner identity, your *roles* vis-à-vis the outside world can fall into place from a clearer perspective.

Step back and reexamine your results from exercises 1, 2, and 3. You have identified your governing values, clarified your most deeply held passions, and embraced your most significant roles. Take some time to let it all settle and digest. You're well on your way to an integrated expression of your sense of purpose.

A brief word is in order here about multitasking and weighing priorities. Juggling multiple roles is never easy. Even when we can pare them down to a manageable number (like Frumma's seven roles), multitasking can challenge a person's ability to know what's *truly* important and what is not.

Greg McKeown, a blogger for the *Harvard Business Review* and the author of *Essentialism*, points out that the word *priorities* was never even seen in the plural form until modern times. People used to focus on one *priority*, and that was it. It'd be a good idea to bear that in mind as you strive to see the unifying thread that runs through all your commitments and become more one-pointed in your life.

You may in fact feel ready now to compose a mission statement or to take a stab at articulating the theme of your Third Act. But hold back just a bit longer. Before we proceed, one more layer of this process is worth a closer look. We're talking about the realm of action, where the rubber hits the road, where all the clarification and introspection and honing of values and intention comes up against that treacherous terrain popularly known as *getting it done.*

Get S.M.A.R.T.

Have you ever had a dream that ended in a rude awakening? How many times in your life have your best intentions amounted to less than expected outcomes? It happens to the best of us. We've discovered that a key turning point lies in the ability to effectively translate intentions into achievable *goals.* Or more precisely, S.M.A.R.T. goals.

If your goals are based on your values and aligned with your passions, you know they're really yours. If they are set forth in recognition of a balanced approach to your various roles in life, you know they will be well received by the people you care about and who care about you. Still, it's entirely possible that you may have trouble meeting your primary goals. No worries; you can apply a simple skill set to solve this problem.

Stephen Covey calls goals "dreams with a deadline." To establish an effective goal plan, he teaches, you need to do four things: (1) write it down; (2) give it a time frame; (3) break it into manageable chunks; and (4) commit.[6]

Approaching this strategy in more precise detail with our coaching clients, we often characterize effective goals with the acronym S.M.A.R.T.

S.M.A.R.T. goals are:

- ✺ **S**pecific: What do I want to accomplish?
- ✺ **M**easurable: How will I know when my goal is accomplished?

- ❧ **A**ttainable: How can the goal be achieved?
- ❧ **R**ealistic: Do I have the necessary resources to get this done?
- ❧ **T**ime-bound: When is the completion of this goal due?

Let's say you have set a specific goal to *write a screenplay*. Does that feel overwhelming? It probably should, because it's not as easy as the average moviegoer might imagine. So you break it down.

- ❧ **Make it more specific.** It's a screenplay based on a short story you wrote in an undergraduate creative writing course.
- ❧ **Make it measurable.** If a saleable screenplay is about 120 pages, you will write x number of pages each week for y number of weeks ($y = 120/x$.)
- ❧ **Make it attainable.** You figure that optimally, on a good week, you can produce 20 solid pages a week.
- ❧ **Make it realistic.** On second thought, given all your other roles and commitments, maybe 10 pages per week is less intimidating. So you've ascertained that $x = 10$ and $y = 12$.
- ❧ **Now make it time-bound.** Pencil in twelve weekly deadlines in your calendar or planner; then block out segments of time for each day during each of those weeks in which to glue yourself to the writing desk and write. Will a holiday or family event somewhere in the middle of those twelve weeks

likely get in the way? Adjust accordingly and reset your schedule.

As a simple illustration, in the accompanying sidebar Frumma focuses on her role as *inspirational speaker* and expresses it in terms of a S.M.A.R.T. goal so that it will evolve from a mere dream into concrete reality. Note that she has written this goal in the present tense to better ensure that it won't be relegated to "someday," or "sometime in the future." She sees herself accomplishing this goal *now*.

You'll want to write down your S.M.A.R.T. goals on a regular basis and track your progress systematically as

....

FRUMMA'S S.M.A.R.T. GOAL

*I am actively working to secure speaking engagements (***specific***), two per month (***measurable***), by committing one hour per week (***attainable***) to email prospective speaking venues.*

*I am composing a speaker's page with a photo, bio, topics and testimonials, to send to each prospect (***realistic***).*

*I am programming an alert on my phone for 10 a.m. every Tuesday (***time-bound***).*

In this way I am achieving my goal: to contract for six new speaking engagements by November 1 of this year.

My core values represented by this goal are community, generosity, leadership, and creativity. I am driven by my passion for coaching people, to help them come unstuck.

....

you proceed. To pursue and achieve your goals more consciously—and therefore with greater, deeper, more consistent commitment—it helps to link them explicitly with the values and passions in which they are rooted, and with the roles associated with them. Write those connections down as well, as Frumma has done here, and as you review your goals from time to time, take a moment to revisit the thought processes and the emotional bonds that gave birth to them.

Putting It All Together: Your Mission Statement

Take a deep breath; let all this introspection and the intention it generates settle in the marrow of your bones. Then write a mission statement that reflects who you are, what you believe in, your strengths and goals, what you love to do, what your gifts to your loved ones will be, and how you would like to be described at the end of this journey.

Some people write their mission statements as poetry. Others compile relevant quotes from famous people. Some are wordy; others manage to articulate the most essential message in a single sentence. You may find it helpful (though it's not necessary) to include specific activities that will help you keep strong and healthy in the physical, emotional, intellectual, and spiritual sectors of your life.

You have now fulfilled the basic prerequisites to composing your mission statement: your dreams have down-to-earth deadlines; you've made room in your busy life for each of your important, cherished roles; your values and your passions have evolved beyond conflict and competition, toward synergy and harmony.

An effective, happy, fulfilled human being is a *whole* human being—one whose mind, heart, capabilities, and intentions are well aligned, one whose arms reach out lovingly toward others and whose legs are long and strong enough to get from here to there. Now, with all your "parts" on the same page and willing to pull together in support of one another, you are finally ready to articulate your mission.

Should you need some assistance, an Internet search will reveal an abundance of tools and sample mission statements online. Keep yours brief, clear, and positive. Rewrite it until it feels good to you. Because it demands deep introspection, it can sometimes take months of crafting before it feels complete.

How will you know? When your mission statement energizes and empowers you rather than overwhelming you, you've probably nailed it.

Now put your mission statement someplace where you can see it. Frame it, or laminate it; emblazon it upon your heart, and revisit it again and again. Seek certainty, but know that absolute certainty will be forever elusive. Be prepared to return to the drawing board when life surprises.

In the sidebars above, Frumma shared some of her own process in defining and crystalizing her roles and goals. The larger sidebar here contains her current mission statement—again, expressed in the present tense. Note how,

FRUMMA'S MISSION STATEMENT

I effectively inspire and empower others and myself toward tangible personal transformation.

I cultivate presence of mind, purposeful habits, social and emotional intelligence, and harmonious relationships.

I practice lovingkindness, respect, compassion, persistence, gratitude, creativity, and joy.

I am receptive to Divine Wisdom and conscious of Divine Unity.

I am a loving wife and an actively engaged matriarch of an extraordinary family.

I continually renew myself by focusing on the four aspects of my life:

Physical: My commitment to daily exercise and healthy eating keeps me strong and well.

Emotional: Through daily meditation, regular entries in my gratitude journal, and intentional choices of positive thoughts and language, I attain inner calm and a trusting temperament, and I make the space to do the things I enjoy.

Intellectual: Through meaningful reading, lectures, and workshops, my knowledge and wisdom grow ever broader and deeper.

Spiritual: The specific blocks of time I devote each day to prayer, learning, and good deeds lead me toward a 24/7 sense of connectedness to Source, expanding awareness, and benevolence toward the world.

I am getting better all the time.

although her statement embodies a number of diverse values, passions, roles, and goals, she envisions herself embracing them all with an overarching, singular sense of purpose.

On to the Next

You achieve the sense of who you are—your *identity*—through becoming more aware of your internal values, passions, and individual strengths. Conversely, your sense of personal *mission* is more about your external commitments and benevolence toward others. These are two distinct aspects of life: *doing*, for the world at large, and *being* who you really are inside.

Some of us are doers—active, energetic extroverts who are all about getting things done. Sometimes that happens at the expense of our own identity, but it happens! On the other hand, some of us accomplish less than we might because we are more introspective, more focused on *being* true to ourselves.

Who is happier, more powerful, better appreciated, more beloved—the introvert or the extrovert? It's a trick question, of course. You can't be yourself without doing for others, and you can't do for others without being yourself. It's the balance between the two, the dance that they do, that makes for a winning mission. The great sage Hillel said it well: "If I am not for myself, who will be for me? And if I am only for myself, who am I? And if not now, when?"[7]

Every mission statement is a work in progress. Chances are you'll be tweaking yours somewhere down the road. Meanwhile, come along with us to chapter 3, into the next dimension of our journey inward and outward, where identity and mission meet.

3

Do Be Do Be Do

Time moves in one direction, memory in another.
—WILLIAM GIBSON

One April morning a few years back, we took a long and leisurely hike along one of the Everglades' swampy trails. We generally prefer mountains to the endlessly flat South Florida terrain, but sometimes you just make the best of what you've got. The hike did not offer spectacular views or much of a workout, but it proved conducive to a certain unperturbed, meditative frame of mind.

At a bend in a creek, a great blue heron stood gracefully still, perched on a fallen log. Most likely a male, to judge by his size and plumage, he seemed at first glance passive, quiescent, the very soul of equanimity. So we too stood still, or as still as humans can stand (which, comparatively, is not all that still). This heron may as well have been made of rock if not for the glint of life in his eye, which shone like a steady flame in a windless place. The only sound was the slight turbulence of the creek and an occasional rustling off in the distance that may have been a rodent, or an alligator—who could know?

Then it happened. At first it was not so much movement as a quickening, a stirring of intention. Then, more suddenly and more powerfully than mere memory can summon up, the heron erupted into action, plunged his head down into the creek, and came up with a fish in his beak. Without a pause he returned as though spring-loaded to his log to enjoy the meal.

We think about this heron every time we come up against that all too human curse of stuckness, of hesitation, of unreadiness to just do what must be done. It's a gap for some, for others an imbalance, between being and doing. Some of us err on the side of impulsive, ill-considered action. Some are so immersed in uncertainty we allow opportunities to slip through our fingers. The heron was fortunate to have no fingers and to know no hesitation; his beak and his stillness and his vigilance and his hunger were entirely one. Though we are human, and therefore given to think before we act and to rethink our actions after the fact, that oneness we saw in a moment of pure movement in the Everglades is an enviable quality.

Two-Way Time Management

Here's a riddle we sometimes use to open up a workshop: five birds are sitting on a tree. Three birds decide to fly away. How many are left on the tree? Simple arithmetic? Not exactly. The correct answer is five. Why? Because there's a big difference between *deciding* and *doing*.

Unless, that is, your decisions emerge seamlessly out of your passionately held values, and fulfill one or more of the roles you've wholeheartedly embraced. In such a case your decisions are simply an expression of who you are. There's no IDD (intention deficit disorder) to stand in the way of your getting it done. Enlightened planning is more than a to-do list; it's a do-be-do-be-do list.

That's why time management tools sell well yet often disappoint. Regardless of which tools we use to effectively manage time, we first need a clear sense of our mission in life, rooted in the values we cherish and focused on the priorities and goals we set. We need to recognize time management as a two-way street, with smooth-flowing traffic back and forth between the inner essence of our identities (who we *be*) and our outer-oriented S.M.A.R.T. goals (what we do and how we do it). If you've been following our suggestions up to this point, you've probably come a long way toward translating your deepest aspirations into skillfully crafted tasks. You may not yet have achieved the primal simplicity of a Tarzan or a hungry heron, but you're on the way.

Choose your planning tool, whether digital or pen-and-ink, desktop or handheld, and prepare to create your schedule. First review your list of roles and then your goals and the approximate time frames you've assigned to them. Make sure a week doesn't go by without scheduling at least a small amount of time to fulfilling every one of your roles. That way you'll stay true to and in touch with all your various relationships, even as you pursue your private, personal visions and dreams.

A schedule is only as good as one's commitment to keep it. And we know (believe us, we *know!*) how fickle commitment can be when the winds of change blow, whether from outside or inside of us. Just because we've drawn our own guidelines and timelines, that doesn't mean we'll toe the line. In fact, for many of us, externally enforced deadlines are *easier* to meet. When there's no gun to our heads, how do we keep from continuously needing to forgive ourselves for falling off the track? (Let's be a little less euphemistic and apply a harsher term: how do we keep from betraying ourselves?)

Here's a secret strategy: each time you pencil in a commitment on your schedule, pause for a moment and trace the task back to its internal origins. What goal does this task serve? Which of your roles is it intended to fulfill? Do you passionately feel its importance? Is this task consistent with your governing values? (Or if it's one of those unpleasant tasks that must be done, can you imagine the delight you'll feel when it's complete?)

Then step all the way back to the big picture: can you see and feel how keeping your commitment for this particular block of time is driven by your mission statement, your abiding sense of purpose?

As you walk through your weeks, consulting the schedule along the way to remind yourself what's next, remember as best you can what each of those to-do items felt like when you were penciling it in. Connect each task at hand to your core. Don't *just* do it. Life is not a Nike ad. Also *be* it. And do, and be, and do, and be. Stride forward into

. . . OR MAYBE NOT?

Does all this cheery talk of goal setting and time management annoy you? It's perfectly understandable for a baby boomer or a retiree to want to say "Enough!—include me out. Leave the visions and the missions for Second-Actors with energy to burn."

For some of us there may be too many hours in the day, too many empty years left. Depression, detachment, or a sense of worthlessness can be very real aspects of advancing years.

If the achievement-oriented exercises here are not quite your cup of tea, that's fine—you'll soon encounter in these pages many paths to tranquility, simplicity, and a quality of life unencumbered by the pressures of "gotta do what you gotta do." You may just discover how letting go of time-bound goals can, paradoxically, help you reclaim a feeling of meaning and purpose in your life.

action even as you step inward and upward in your memory of who you are. Connect the dots between whatever you're up to just now and the emotions, perspectives, and intentions that brought you here.

Time Affluence

No discussion of calendars and planners would be complete without a deeper look at the meaning of time itself. Time is the one commodity in life that, once wasted, can never be reclaimed. When we're young, we think we have all the time in the world; as we mature and become better attuned to our mortality, the preciousness of time looms larger. There are only so many moments in an hour, so many hours in a day, so many years remaining before we move on to . . . well, let's not have that conversation just now.

There's a phrase bouncing around of late in the literature of positive psychology that, though newly fashionable, evokes the wisdom of the ancients. The expression is *affluence of time*. It conveys a sense of abundance rather than scarcity, a sense that we have all the time we need rather than being pressed for time or worrying that there's not enough time to do what must be done.

How do we acquire that consciousness? On the surface, time is obviously finite. "Gotta hurry, behind schedule, jammed up, stressed and overworked, sorry, no time, I'm exhausted!" Sound familiar? These protestations are an inevitable result of perceiving "blocks of time" as though each hour is the same as any other hour. A deeper, more profound perspective is available, however, that sees every moment as unique, and in a sense infinite.

About nine hundred years ago in medieval Spain there lived a poet, philosopher, and Bible scholar by the name of Abraham ibn Ezra. Though he struggled all his life to make ends meet (he used to say that if he were in the business of making funeral shrouds, people would stop dying), his wisdom was extraordinary and relevant to this day. (There was some light back in those so-called dark ages!) His short poem, freely translated here, provides a key to achieving affluence of time:

The past is naught.
The future? Not yet.
The present—like the blink of an eye.
Should one then worry? Why?[8]

Today's quantum physicists tend to agree. They speak about the "unreality" of time as we generally understand it, and how the only unit of time that truly exists is this very instant, now. Kabbalists, the mystics of Judaism, carry it a step further with the doctrine of continuous creation, declaring that the entire universe is actually coming into existence anew every moment—and that the way human beings behave in this moment influences the way the universe is made. Like many other beautiful, potentially life-changing ideas, this is not the way we generally tend to think. But it's not all that complicated.

One coach we've worked with introduced us to a quick but effective shortcut to such presence of mind. We often suggest it to our clients and patients. It takes just three deep breaths. We've placed it in a sidebar (next page) for easy future reference.

Though it's a breathing exercise, this does not call for any exertion or forcing of the breath, as some breathing exercises require. Keep it relaxed, almost effortless. By allowing a power beyond you to breathe through you, you will have gotten yourself and your anxieties out of the way. It's no longer about you and your limitations. It's a mini-vacation of sorts, a small Sabbath. You've just gone from zero to infinity in sixty seconds.

A ONE-MINUTE MEDITATION

Take a full breath, filling your lungs, chest, and abdomen. Inhale, then exhale, and with that exhale release any lingering attachments, concerns, or regrets associated with things that have happened in the past.

Inhale a second time, and then exhale and release all your fears or worries about the future.

Then take a third deep breath, and as you exhale easily, allow yourself to be fully aware of the limitless creative potential emerging from within you in this present moment.

For those inevitable stressful times when breathing easy is anything but, it's still simple enough to harness the power of this moment, this blink of an eye. All it takes is a straight-ahead good deed. Let your next action be an act of kindness. Not a "random act of kindness," as the popular slogan goes, but rather an *intentional* deed, based on your best assessment of how you can improve the situation in front of your face. Change a light bulb. Wash a dish. Pick up someone's litter. And recognize that you are participating in the rectification of the world. Which is actually the re-*creation* of the world.

Take it a step further: Can you make a close friend or relation a little happier, a little more optimistic, a little closer to his or her goal? OK, maybe you can't *make* her happy; only she can accomplish that. But there's something you can do to make her life a little easier. What's your best next step? Do it now, and pay attention to its purpose now.

You might also avail yourself of a little technological assistance. A timer, such as the one on most cell phones, can help you wholeheartedly occupy the "now." Once you've decided that a given twenty minutes is going to be spouse time, or best-friend time, or writing or exercise or squandering-time-on-the-Internet time, set the timer. Begin when it begins and end when it ends. Get into whatever it is you are doing 100 percent, and don't think about whatever else is on the schedule until the timer says, "On to the next." Right now, you are all spouse, all friend, all dad, or all grandma. By being fully present in that role, we magnify empathy and passion and solidify commitment.

We live in a world of external distraction, surrounded by devices that beep, tweet, toot, and tout the urgency of the next spurious demand on our time and attention. Even the cozy niches where we used to go to enjoy quality time are plastered with flashing screens evoking silent screams. To be fully present, we have to rein ourselves in.

An acquaintance of ours, an international speaker who had been away from home on tour for ten days, wanted to do something special with his children to make up for his absence. He decided to take them out to dinner. So he asked them if they wanted Italian, Chinese, or the local burgers/fries emporium. To which his six-year-old son replied, "I don't really care, I just want you!"

Life is a walking meditation, and your presence is requested. In other words, if we are able to cultivate presence of mind, if we genuinely possess the present moment and live fully in the now, then we really do have all the time in the world. This is time affluence.

Material affluence, of course, can't buy happiness; neither can an abundance of time. Although psychological research has demonstrated that time affluence (unlike material wealth) can be a strong predictor of well-being, it is far from a guarantee. Time can be our greatest asset or our worst enemy. Use it well, infuse each moment with purposefulness, and we are in flow. Fritter it away, and we are in pain.

Sanctifying Time: Rituals and Habit-Stacking

Some of us are loath to admit it, but deep within the nooks and crannies of the human mind lives a powerful desire for orderliness, stability, compliance with a consistent schedule. It's a fact of nature that the sun and the moon whirl and twirl their ways through years and months with stunning regularity; that seasons and sunsets display a fascinating but predictable rhythm; that bodies perform best when they rest and rise at the same time from day to day.

The same is true of souls. Chaos confines us; constancy frees us. Like zucchinis, begonias, and hundred-year-old oak trees, our talents and achievements are best grown gradually, incrementally. Sudden spurts of energy and creativity will inevitably be punctuated by crashes, sluggishness, and downtime. They rarely get the big jobs done.

Time affluence liberates us from a sense of pressure and anxiety. It allows us to pursue meaningful activities in the service of our life's mission. But to make the most of our time, to gain proactive mastery of time, to become the *cause* rather than the *effect* in the fulfillment of our intentions, we need to learn how to sanctify time. Has the sun ever refused to rise just because it doesn't feel up to it? If we want to become that reliable, we need to behave as though hardwired with an inexorable sense of purpose. This is a key component of the art of *getting better all the time.* And to this end, there is no more effective tool in our toolbox than the judicious use of ritual.

Rituals are very precise behaviors, performed at specific times and motivated by deeply held values. They support our higher purpose, and they are nonnegotiable. For example, even though we might not have grown up flossing our teeth, we floss in the morning and/or evening. It has become automatic because we have bought into the concept that reducing plaque makes for a healthier mouth (and, research suggests, a healthier heart).[9]

Rituals support our goals and visions by incorporating actions into our *everyday* life, not just our *someday,* want-to-be life. Far from stifling us with rigid behaviors, rituals actually facilitate inspiration. Harvard University's Dr. Tal Ben Shahar addressed this idea in his best-selling book *Happier*: "The most creative individuals—whether artists, businesspeople, or parents—have rituals that they follow. Paradoxically, the routine frees them up to be creative and spontaneous."[10]

We are what we repeatedly do.
Excellence, then, is not an act, but a habit.
—ARISTOTLE

In their book *The Power of Full Engagement*, performance coaches Jim Loehr and Tony Schwarz explain: "Initiating a ritual is often difficult, but maintaining it is relatively easy. Top athletes have rituals: they know that at specific hours during each day they are on the field, after which they are in the gym, and then they stretch. . . . We need to take the same approach toward any change we want to introduce."[11]

What sort of rituals would make you happier, more purposeful, more energetic and effective? What would you like to introduce into your life? It could be exercising three times a week, meditating for ten minutes every morning, going on a date with your spouse on Tuesday evenings, reading for pleasure for an hour every other day. Once you identify a ritual you want to adopt, enter it in your planner and begin to keep the commitment.

New rituals may be difficult in the beginning, so keep them short and simple at first, and introduce no more than one or two rituals at a time. Before very long, usually within as little as thirty days, performing these rituals will become as natural as brushing your teeth. Make sure each ritual becomes a habit before you introduce a new one. Habits are generally difficult to break; with good habits, that's good news.

THE GRATITUDE JOURNAL

Here's a ritual you'll be glad you made a part of your life: keep a daily gratitude journal. A plethora of evidence has shown the benefits of this practice. In their book *The Psychology of Gratitude*, Robert Emmons and Michael McCullough describe a study whose participants were simply told to write down five things for which they were grateful every day. Those who kept a gratitude journal enjoyed remarkably higher levels of emotional and physical well-being.[12]

Try it yourself and feel the difference in your life. Each night before going to sleep, write down at least five things you appreciate. They can be little or big, from a meal you enjoyed to a meaningful conversation you had with a friend, from a project successfully completed at work to sublime gratitude toward God. Consider what each item means to you as you write it down; experience the feeling associated with it. Doing this exercise regularly can transform the tone of your life. It will train you not just to appreciate but also to anticipate and discover positive aspects of life that you might miss when you're in the habit of taking things for granted.

Your first thoughts of the day are powerful. Those early waking moments are a perfect time for acknowledging the restoration of your soul from the torpor of sleep and the fatigue of the night before. First thing in the morning, as you emerge into awareness, establish a relationship with the source of your life as you understand it. Whether it's a simple expression of thanks or a thoughtful contemplation of the Creator, gratitude helps us form a sense of connection. We can then take a moment to ask for guidance through the day, in choosing positive, purposeful thoughts and actions and steering clear of selfishness, resentment, and envy.

A parallel practice is useful before we go to sleep. Whereas most hours of most days are best spent being present in the moment (and perhaps looking ahead), bedtime is one of those few occasions when it is helpful to look back in a frank assessment of our day. Take note of shortcomings: lapses in judgment; betrayal of trust; unnecessary anger; an overcritical eye upon loved ones and colleagues; feelings of bitterness or victimization. Then—and this is important (in fact it's the point!)—we can reach deep within to forgive ourselves and others. From that place of forgiveness, we can effectively resolve to make amends where needed—and sleep more soundly to boot.

With the day well bracketed with morning and evening introspection, you've cleared the decks a bit; it becomes easier to hone your intentions throughout the day. As you proceed further along in this book, you'll find any number of nourishing practices that you might choose to adopt or adapt as your personal rituals. Choose wisely; consider your personal priorities, according to your self-determined goals and roles. Be sure to reserve the best hours of your days for the activities you deem most important. If being a potter is number one on your hit parade, take care to designate time at the potter's wheel when you are energized and feeling your best. Unless you are Martha Stewart, don't use your prime productive time for shopping or cooking or cleaning.

STACKING YOUR DECK

Remember that growth happens incrementally. It can be tempting to pile on the positive practices and find yourself overwhelmed with a long list of musts and shoulds. For some of us, surrendering the busyness of a forty-year career leaves us grieving, and anxious to rapidly replace the emptiness before we become has-beens in our own minds. A morning devoted to exercise, meditation, journaling, prayer, sipping a hot cup of freshly squeezed lemon tea, and plowing through an indispensable and ever-expanding list of required reading might seem ideal, but could prove too much too soon. Keep it small and simple in the beginning, with sustainable five-minute time slots that grow gradually and multiply with care and caution. Try the habit-stacking exercise outlined on the next page. Before long, you will have your own customized set of meaningful rituals that nourish and structure your days.

Optimally, your habit stack will take precedence over other obligations. The sense of routine and rhythm you will achieve will quiet the mind, send healthy messages to your body, and enhance creativity. Inevitably, there will be situations when you'll need to adjust to unusual demands on your time, perhaps by breaking up the schedule into two or more sessions. Conversely, there will be days when you feel so inspired, enthused, or rippling with discipline that you'll want to keep a particular ritual spinning beyond the allotted time. We humbly suggest that you learn to resist such temptation. Give this slow, small method a chance to succeed. Like the fabled terrapin of Aesop's fable "The Tortoise and the Hare," you will watch yourself arrive at the finish line in triumph thanks to the slow and steady approach.

THE HABIT STACK

If introducing one purposeful ritual is a good idea, imagine the benefit of constructing a meaningful daily regimen of several practices that cover all the bases, from physical health to spiritual well-being and back again—a stack of habits that make getting better all the time as consistently a part of you as washing your face in the morning. It's possible, if you embrace this process. The key is to methodically link together small, easily accomplished, routine practices that naturally belong together.

1. Choose two, and only two, rituals or disciplines that you know will contribute to your happiness, health, or success if you do them each day. Yoga? Swimming? Prayer? Abdominal crunches? Learning a new language? Sunbathing or stargazing? Whichever two work for you, and which logically enhance each other or go together back-to-back.

2. Establish a time at which you can do these practices each day, and stick with it. It may be first thing in the morning, when the birds are chirping, or a late evening routine, when the world is likely to leave you in peace. If you can stick with a consistent starting time, at least for the first month, your stack will have more staying power.

3. Limit the allotted time: do your two activities for only five minutes each. Does that seem too laid-back or self-indulgent? No! You're not a wimp. You're guaranteeing you won't spin out. You're astutely easing into excellence.

4. Make a daily commitment, make it nonnegotiable, and show up. If you miss a day, don't quit, and certainly don't beat yourself up; just try to return to your intention as quickly as possible.

5. Add one minute to each activity each week. Yes, just one minute per week: trust us, it'll add up. If your week proved too difficult to add a minute to your habit stack, stick with the same number of minutes for another week. Be sure to take a moment to praise yourself for showing up!

6. When you are ready (meaning solid and comfortable in your new habit stack), add another activity instead of another minute. Then repeat the weekly increase of one minute per practice.

7. Continue the process of gradually acclimating and adding activities and minutes until you have a stack of habits that makes you feel powerful, flourishing, and delighted with your ongoing progress. You might stop and stabilize at thirty minutes or ninety minutes; it's your call. Listen attentively to what your newly attuned intuition tells you.

As we advance in years, energy becomes an increasingly cherished commodity. We commonly expect that as our clocks and calendars pick up their pace, we'll have less energy than back in the day. On a purely biological level, that may be true. Physicists tell us, however, that globally, galactically, conservation of energy rules. The energy may have relocated or regrouped—may in fact seem to elude us—but it hasn't disappeared. We can gain access to that unflagging font of potential power. We can give ourselves a boost simply by lining up our actions and intentions with the essence of who we really are and what we truly want.

In fact, we may discover that we have more energy than ever in the Third Act of our lives, because we're finally galvanizing and integrating all the scattered, incoherent energy that we were only barely aware we had. We had limitless vigor, or so it seemed, in our younger years, and happily, we managed to put much of it to work. But the true power was stored offline in latent memory, like the untapped amperage of a forgotten storage battery. Now we've become aware that the most effective connection is a wireless one, and we know the code.

∽ ∽ ∽ ∽ ∽

In Part One we have focused on defining ourselves, articulating our life's purpose. We have outlined the milestones of our Third Acts, envisioned the arcs of our stories, and taken possession of the tools we've acquired over a lifetime of learning.

Part Two is more devoted to the internal development of character. We'll explore, in loving detail, the refinement and alignment of heart, mind, and soul that will empower us to bring our mission statements to fruition.

*The whole is greater than
the sum of its parts.*

—ARISTOTLE

PART TWO

Diversity is one of those buzzwords everyone seems to agree about
until they start discussing what it really means. "*E pluribus unum,*"
the American motto proudly proclaims: "*Out of many, one.*"
Turns out it's a tough row to hoe. We'll leave the societal
implications to politicians and social scientists; here we're
interested in the microcosm. What do diversity and
oneness mean within each of us personally?

We are complex and sometimes conflicted individuals.
We are made of mind and heart, body and soul, ambition
and escapism, love and fear. How do we pull all that
together and become whole?

Part Two offers a detailed map of the interior landscape of the
human personality—a practical guide to exploring all our inner
mountaintops, swamps, back alleys and six-lane highways—with
an eye toward integrating our disparate parts. The goal is to
establish and maintain optimal efficacy and wellness: mentally,
emotionally, spiritually, and physically.

PART TWO

4

Revisiting Spirituality

*Nothing is inherently and invincibly young except spirit.
And spirit can enter a human being perhaps better
in the quiet of old age, and dwell there more
undisturbed than in the turmoil of adventure.*

—GEORGE SANTAYANA

There's a classic American show tune that captures both the challenge of growing older and its cure. The song has been performed over many decades by such a long and diverse list of artists—from Paul Robeson, Frank Sinatra, and Ray Charles to Al Jolson, Screamin' Jay Hawkins, and the Beach Boys—it must be meaningful. It first appeared in the 1929 Broadway musical *Showboat*, with music by Jerome Kern and lyrics by Oscar Hammerstein II. To this day, you can no doubt hear it echoing somewhere in the back of your mind:

> *Ah gits weary*
> *An' sick of tryin'*
> *Ah'm tired of livin'*

An' skeered of dyin',
But Ol' Man River
He jes' keeps rollin' along.

We all have moments when we feel tired, over the hill, or headed inexorably downstream. But if we can step back and see the big picture, the river redeems us. There's something rejuvenating, something *spiritual* about a river. It just keeps rollin' along, flowing from the mountaintops down to the sea, watering farmlands along its path, then returning and recirculating through clouds and rainfall in the never-ending cycle of life.

Whether or not that's what the good Mr. Hammerstein had in mind, the fact is that Ol' Man River has a way of making us feel young. Nothing refreshes the spirit quite so delightfully as a twenty-minute interlude, propped up against a tree by a babbling brook. It's a perfect setting for a meditation or a daydream. Flowing waters seem to free us from our stuck places and disentangle us from anxieties or regrets.

It makes sense culturally and historically as well. Countless traditions have conveyed spiritual significance through the image of the river. Hermann Hesse's *Siddhartha* recounts the story of the young Indian prince who sat by the river Ganges in meditative grace until he achieved enlightenment and became a Buddha.

The patriarch Abraham's journey began in Mesopotamia, between the Tigris and Euphrates rivers, and culminated in his crossing the Jordan into the Promised Land. In the Western Hemisphere too, the Mississippi, the Shenandoah, the Rio Grande, and the Amazon loom larger than life in the minds and the myths of men.

In the Flow

In the dynamics of the flowing stream, we find meaning, purpose, and power. The massive hydroelectric power harnessed by a Hoover Dam is an obvious example, but it's in the small tributaries that we discover a more personal, more intimate energy. A classic parable tells the tale of a certain great scholar who was ignorant and unaccomplished until he was forty years of age. Then one day he observed how the trickle of water from a tiny rivulet had, over time, worn a gigantic hole in a boulder. In that steady drip-drip-drip he realized the greatness of his own potential, if he would just keep on keeping on.

Physical strength is rooted in spiritual strength, and both are about flow. Great athletes speak about being *in the zone* of peak performance; happiness and creativity are maximized when we are so fully immersed in what we're doing, so dynamically in the moment, that all distractions and concerns slip away. It was a famous Hungarian-American professor of psychology with the unpronounceable name of Mihaly Csikszentmihalyi (unspellable too, without a little help) who first identified this ideal state of nonstop focused awareness as *flow*.

On the simplest level, the professor explains, it makes us feel good to be unselfconsciously engaged in whatever activity is at hand. It promotes physical health as well. Physical well-being, as we'll discuss in greater detail in chapter 14, is a function of being whole, of feeling wholly connected with every aspect of our internal and external environment. A healthy physical body becomes a ready, receptive vessel for spiritual flow, bringing us exhilaration, inspiration, the joy of being wholly alive. We are open, excited, awake, and alert, delighted and surprised by the simple, amazing presence of everything that exists.[13]

Rivers, great places to hang out for a while on a crisp autumn afternoon, provide us with potent metaphysical metaphors as well. The sages and masters of many inner disciplines speak of human consciousness as a *stream* that emerges from the depths of our soul's essence, then extends downstream to water all our activities and make all our endeavors grow. The *river* represents unobstructed flow from our spiritual source all the way through to our down-to-earth everyday experiences. So while this is not the place for an in-depth discussion of the mystical dimensions of connecting to "spiritual source" (whatever that may mean to you), there's a good reason why we decided to deal with this subject of spirituality before tackling the mental, emotional, and active behavioral aspects of aging. If we're going to get in the groove and go with the flow, it's a good idea to have some sense of where the flow is coming from.

When we speak of spirituality, we mean it in an utterly nonsectarian sense, untethered to any particular belief system, doctrine, or religious institution. Not that we are unaffiliated ourselves. We identify proudly with a tradition that harks back to revelation at Sinai and looks forward confidently toward a future characterized by universal brotherhood and love. Many of the principles we've gleaned from our studies are universally applicable and resonate with truths expressed in other traditions. We present them here, to the best of our ability, in ways that will be useful to all readers.

In these interesting, diverse, turbulent times, some people are uncomfortable with the G-word. They may prefer to refer to a less personal Oneness, or to the Universe, or the Force (thanks, Yoda!)—or to no transcendent entity at all. You may or may not see yourself as a believer in a singular deity. You may or may not have cultivated a relationship with a Higher Power; perhaps you view the world through the lens of natural law. (Some of us worship the car-key God, as in: "Oh, God, where are my car keys?") We're not inclined to argue about it. We figure that men and women of good will can find ways to work together and inspire one another, and that eventually "truth will sprout forth from the earth" (Psalm 85:11).

Our confidence is rooted in experience. Nature has a way of suggesting that there's something going on beyond the limits of natural phenomena. We've seen how, if one is willing to step back and take a broader perspective, there's a sense of underlying unity even in the midst of the incredible diversity of this material world. Even where conflict is most obvious, a potential resolution seems to lurk just behind the curtain.

FRUMMA CONFESSES

I grew up with a Park Avenue education, full-time domestic help, and a silver spoon. It was only natural that my default mode tended to be a tad materialistic. There have been many moments when the desire for a new car with leather upholstery and state-of-the-art audio, a charming country estate with horses and weather vanes, or the latest fashion from Bergdorf's, would rob me of my peace of mind. A shame, because between kids' tuition payments, a life punctuated with carpools and diaper changes, and the ups and downs of multiple careers, not much luxury was likely. (These days the diapers are only worn by grandchildren. I get to change them on a discretionary basis, albeit with great gusto.)

According to conventional wisdom, materialism is spirituality's polar opposite. I beg to differ. I do not buy the notion that the spiritual life demands austerity. Perhaps that was once the case, but not today. Allow me to point out that God is not merely spiritual, any more than He is physical. Yes, it's certainly liberating to have mostly outgrown the old passionate need for luxury. It frees up a lot of my energy to expand my mind and heart and cultivate relationships with the Infinite. But I am still a big fan of the material world, albeit with a bit more equanimity, a lot less entitlement, and an evolving sense that what's mine may just as well be yours. All aspects of existence, including this material world, are expressions of divine delight.

Our generation was schooled early on in such paradigm shifts. In 1972, we saw the first full photograph of planet Earth viewed from space, taken by the Apollo 17 astronauts. Suddenly, local reality became a little less real. From that point on, global, whole-earth consciousness was no longer just an esoteric idea; oneness had become visible, tangible, almost a no-brainer.

> *There are only two ways to live your life.*
> *One is as though nothing is a miracle.*
> *The other is as though everything is a miracle.*
> —ALBERT EINSTEIN

Just as that sense of harmonious possibility was revealed then in the cosmos, so is it emerging today in the way we understand the microcosm. Through a whole-systems approach to human health and an integral model of human psychology, we are redefining what it means to be well. It means being unfragmented, complete. It's a recognition that we are far more than merely the sum our parts, and that we are capable of overcoming apparent conflicts among our various parts with a single courageous quantum leap. This may not look like spirituality in the conventional sense. It's not religiosity, and it does not demand faith up front.

We've seen, however, that cultivating creativity and integrity in our worldly activities invites in spirituality and nourishes a certain kind of faith. Not blind faith, but an internalized awareness that we are *so* small, and reality is infinite . . . and accessible.

Cultivating Spiritual Intelligence

Consider the classic conflict between the head and the heart. We know very well what we *ought to* love, but we love things we shouldn't. We understand when there's no reason to be afraid, but we're terrified anyway. "How could something so wrong feel so right?" And so on. There are methods of developing emotional intelligence that can help sort out such internal battles (see chapter 6). These methods are largely based on the understanding that the mind and the emotions are intertwined, that we can discern the seeds of our feelings in our intellect, and vice versa, and adjust accordingly.

Practically speaking, however, our various parts can prove stubborn. That's where emotional intelligence can fail. It doesn't necessarily cure all our meltdowns. We also need to be connected on a level that transcends the limitations of our hearts and our heads: spiritual intelligence to the rescue.

Spiritual intelligence does not, alas, confer sainthood upon us. No matter how much wiser we get as we age, plenty of battles remain. Egos will still flare their nostrils. Fists will more than likely clench from time to time. We may still hunger insatiably for superficial signs of validation or approval from outside ourselves. But with increasing access to dimensions of the spirit, the odds will be tweaked in our favor. In our Third Act of life, we can finally acquire the wisdom to look inward rather than outward for applause or acclaim.

A story is told about a famous eighteenth-century spiritual leader, frail and well on in years, who was able to navigate an icy, steep, and slippery mountain pass with little effort. His younger, stronger disciples, following close behind, found the treacherous climb an enormous challenge. Upon finally reaching the peak, they asked him how he had kept his footing with such ease and grace. "If a man is connected on high," he replied, "he doesn't fall down below."

We have mountains to climb and miles to go. Having honed our mission statements to become and achieve everything we've envisioned, we'll want to cultivate spiritual intelligence. Whether we have some grand plan or simply desire to live each day to the fullest, it will serve us well to bind ourselves on high, lest we stumble and fall.

In the next several chapters we'll be looking at the various interconnected aspects of the human personality—intellect, emotions, speech, and deed—with an eye toward integrating all our disparate parts and maintaining optimal health physically, emotionally, and mentally.

Then, in Part Three, we'll turn our attention outward toward a sense of service and agency in the world at large. We'll focus on the many levels of our relationships with spouses, families, and communities, and on the quality of life we convey, the gifts we give, the legacies we'll leave. Spiritual intelligence drives and guides this journey, culminating in behavioral intelligence. In the coming chapters, we will offer training in some of the methods that have worked for us and present tools that will help you discover and activate your own best intentions.

You will inevitably run into low points and high points along the way. Down in the trenches, we'll do our best to heal wounds, bring comfort to broken hearts, and rectify what's gone wrong. And up in the heights of sublime experience, good will get better and pleasure will become more and more refined, drawing from divine delight, not for your own self-gratification, but for the sake of sharing.

None of this is attainable or sustainable if we rely solely on our own innate expertise, cleverness, or compassion. To be in flow is to catch a wave that's way bigger than we are. The surest way to get better all the time is to learn to defer to a wisdom greater than our own, a power greater than ourselves. Like Tarzan swinging from vine to vine, we need to practice the art of letting go and moving on. The process is based on trust, but it is balanced with commitment, perseverance, responsibility, and accountability. Connection to a Higher Power, however we define it, will keep us on an even keel and flying freely through the trees.

· ·

A PERSONAL JOURNEY

We became curious about spirituality in the 1960s. What intrigued us initially was primarily the feeling of mental clarity and physical well-being that accrued from experimenting with such practices as zazen, yoga, and macrobiotic diets. Organic gardening and wilderness living deepened our relationship with nature; meditation piqued our interest in dimensions of life that transcend (and enrich) the natural world. One of our mentors in those early years, an author of cookbooks with poetic, philosophical overtones, would frequently speak about the natural progression, as human beings mature, "from the biological to the spiritual." It rang true.

Another mentor, a teacher of meditation from India, advised us to "consult the scriptures of our birth" in order to integrate spiritual sensibilities with practical daily life. There was something in our own backyard, long ignored, that proved to be surprisingly accessible, that offered a sense of familiarity and, eventually, destiny. We began to explore and embrace values that are eternal and absolute, yet subject to a healthy measure of customized interpretation. The resulting sense of focus and security served to enhance and deepen our concept of individual purpose and communal responsibility.

Prayer and study became daily commitments; an intimate relationship with our Higher Power became our most fertile resource. It's seen us through some pretty hard times: financial issues, challenges to physical and mental health, bankruptcy, and divorce. Having grappled with a fair share of uncertainty and doubt along the way, we've come to trust that everything in life happens for a reason, that we won't be given a test larger than we can handle, and that the dominant energy in the universe is boundless, unconditional benevolence. You might call that faith, but at this stage of the game, it feels more like common sense. As such, it leaves us with a clear memory of where we're coming from and a great deal of respect for the sometimes differing perspectives of our friends.

5

Life of the Mind

Think well, and all will be well.

—HASIDIC APHORISM

It's been said that it takes about a hundred years for a new idea to take root and bear fruit in the minds and hearts of humankind. Case in point: the early twentieth-century development of quantum physics. We're approaching that hundred-year mark about now.

At first, quantum theory's fantastic, improbable predictions were met with skepticism. Though there are still pockets of resistance, after some outside-the-box research experiments, even old-school scientists have begun to take it seriously. But the real proof of its acceptance can be seen in the popular culture: self-help gurus, always on the prowl for quick-fix solutions to our deepest yearnings, have managed to oversimplify and exaggerate its principles. The trendy idea of a law of attraction has made its way into airport bookstore best sellers and the sort of magazines we find at supermarket checkout counters. So it seems we're nearly ready to apply quantum theory to our lives in a meaningful and sustainable way.

One of the originators of quantum physics, Werner Heisenberg, suggested with his uncertainty principle that the perception of an observer can alter what he sees. Today the notion that our outer reality is influenced by our inner mindset has begun to gain favor. It may not be absolutely true that we "create our own reality," but the way we see definitely affects what we get.

So for purely practical reasons, we want to learn how to navigate the landscape of consciousness. For that we'll need a trail map. It's a jungle in there.

The average person has between 65,000 and 75,000 thoughts a day. The bad news is that up to 80 percent of those thoughts are weighed down with some negative content, if they are not altogether negative. We are all plagued by anxieties and fear, anger and grief, or a carping, relentless inner critic. The Internet hasn't helped, keeping us informed of tragedies and injustices all over the world within minutes of their occurrence. And there is no lack of roadblocks and blunders in our personal lives that can produce a steady stream of insecure thoughts if left unchecked.

Negative thoughts flow easily and reverberate repeatedly because they are infused with adrenaline. When we are threatened or attacked or lost, when we've made some terrible mistake or have simply forgotten something important, we react by going into fight-or-flight mode. Our heartbeat accelerates, our breathing becomes shallower, our muscles and blood vessels constrict. We are uptight. A wounded ego cries out, "Why am I so stupid? Why do these things always happen to me?" Our physical responses to the drama act like an indelible highlighter on that unlucky moment in life. That's why we tend to remember feelings of inadequacy far more easily than we can recall our general state of competency.

Today's science, however, is reassuring. The happy buzzword is *neuroplasticity*, which means that the brain is not an impenetrable black box—we can *change* our minds. We can become more selective with our thoughts, rearrange the paths they travel on, and thereby transform our lives.

Ah, but how, when the odds seem so stacked against us? Of those tens of thousands of daily thoughts, upwards of 90 percent are the same thoughts that plagued us yesterday!

The next few chapters will present a number of strategic approaches to achieving and reinforcing neuroplasticity and applying the changes in our lives.

Parts of the Brain, Aspects of the Mind

On a simplistic physiological level, our brain is composed of a series of compartments with different jobs. The lowest level is the *amygdala* (or "lizard brain") adjacent to the brain stem. This section of the brain, charged with protecting us and keeping us safe, is the epicenter of our reactive fight-or-flight mode of thinking. It derives its material from habitual behavior, fondly known as the instinctual, uncultivated inner child. The lizard brain is fast-firing and fast-responding. It is also the area of the brain that serves as our autopilot when we rely, for better or for worse, on same-old-same-old, well-worn habitual patterns. At such times the inner child can lose some of its charm and behave more like an inner brat.

Higher-level modes of thinking take place in the *cerebral cortex*, up closer to the top of the skull. Its intellectual inventory consists of all the ethical and philosophical ideas, historical or scientific theories and data, and cultural values to which we have been exposed throughout our lives, whether at the dinner table, in graduate school, or in houses of worship. Stimuli make their way up to and circulate through this more sophisticated thought bank a bit more slowly. We don't count on this area to be the first responder in an emergency. It does, however, supply us with conceptual inspiration for living a higher, more value-driven existence—that is, when the amygdala isn't busy hijacking its train of thought.

This book is not the place for exploring in detail the rapidly evolving findings of neuroscience. However, we will, in the next chapter on emotional intelligence, present at least one method of mediating between the lizard brain and the higher mind—something we call "wait training." But let's first have a look at a somewhat different, though complementary, map of the mind. It should serve us well in our intention to gain mastery over our minds and influence our world.

The mystics often employ metaphors to render abstract ideas more accessible to concrete thinkers. As we've seen in the previous chapter, one of their most useful metaphors is the concept of the *stream* of consciousness, likened to a river that flows from its source to nourish life downstream. Examined more closely, it offers us a comprehensive overview of the dynamics of the human mind, according to a kabbalistic model.

Where do ideas come from? Where were they before they occurred to us? How does a fleeting, elusive glimmer of insight develop into a full-fledged thought that can be communicated to another? By what magic does the associative mind draw parallels and contrasts and fetch seemingly unrelated notions from afar to dance together and sing new songs? (Einstein called this sort of creative imagination "combinatory play.") The secrets are in the stream.

The Stream of Consciousness

Deep below the surface of the earth, still waters are gathered, unperturbed and unrevealed. In the analog of consciousness, this is the realm of latent intellect. It is thought before we think it, knowledge before we know it. In these subterranean conduits, subconscious processes prepare to bring thoughts to the surface. Then the waters find an opening and emerge in the trickle of a spring high up in the hills. This is the first flash of an idea piercing through to the conscious mind. Like those first drops of the spring, it is pure and pristine. But it may not go far, because this initial impulse of a new idea is still immature, undeveloped. Only when the spring gathers momentum and breadth, becoming first a brook, then a stream, and finally a mighty river does it grow strong and voluminous enough to irrigate farmland, generate power, and build a civilization. The fully developed idea gains momentum and potential as it wends its way downstream. Once an intuitive flash that was meaningful only to its owner, it is now a clear, well-elucidated concept—maybe even a curriculum or a business plan—with core principles and practical applications that other thinkers and doers can consider, critique, and put to work.

On the other hand, the stream has also picked up some turbulence, muck, and mire along the way. The waters of the mighty river far downstream are never as pure as the mountain spring at its source. What once seemed true and simple can become complicated, confusing, corrupt. To get it right and keep it real, the seeker of truth may need to retrace the steps of her thinking back to their source. Imagine a mind that can develop complex ideas in great detail, with the analytical sophistication it takes to invent new technologies or solve pressing problems—yet can at the same time sustain the pristine clarity, simplicity, and tranquility of a quiet spring giving birth to original vision.

Harnessing the Power of the Mind

One of the pillars of aging well is the ability to cultivate a deeper, clearer, more powerful mind. With this metaphor in hand, we can discover new ways to enhance the quality of our cognitive faculties and become effective agents of change. (Not to mention remembering where we left the car keys.) No metaphor is perfect, of course; many aspects of the way minds work call for other sorts of explanation. But this concept of the stream of consciousness (what we've offered here is a simplified version) gives us plenty to work with. It provides a model whereby we can gauge how effectively we're using our minds. Again, the benchmark we've found useful here is to evaluate to what extent the downstream power of the mind is consciously connected to its upstream source.

There's a lot to be said for the "use it or lose it" school of mental exercise. All other things being equal, the more we study, discuss, and contemplate ideas that pique our interest, the less likely we are to become forgetful, dull, or intellectually lazy. Take a course; join a book club; get involved in an online forum or study group. Information is nourishing. The more challenging the subject matter, the better—provided that the content is not so over your head that it's beyond your comfort zone.

> *Life moves fast. If you don't stop and look*
> *around once in a while you could miss it.*
> —FERRIS BUELLER

This sort of in-depth study, however, as stimulating and uplifting as it may be, generally takes place far downstream. In a busy mind, it's easy to lose the purity and tranquility of the deep source of the stream. As a result, our thought processes may be characterized by turbulence and confusion. One factor that helps immeasurably is to be selective about the sorts of information we absorb. Reading in-depth analyses of the global crises of the hour may be compelling in a rather adrenaline-fueled way, but the quality of life it engenders can't compare to delving into the great works of literature, philosophy, poetry, scripture, and wisdom. One of the ubiquitous catchphrases of the 1960s was "feed your head." Let's not forget how this slogan jibes with another popular one from the same period: "You are what you eat." So be selective. Tip: don't watch the news before going to sleep.

Optimally, consuming the right material and digesting it well will enlighten and refine our minds. Contemplating the words of great sages whose streams of consciousness were broad and deep will tend to evoke a similar breadth and depth in us. Nonetheless, listening to Mozart doesn't get you a gig in Carnegie Hall. If you really want to become all that you can be, if the pursuit of excellence is part of your game plan, if you want your intellect to play a starring role in the thrilling climax of your Third Act, you might just need some practice. Let's look at a few fascinating ways to exercise the mind.

Meditation for ~~Dummies~~ Geniuses

Practices that cultivate mindfulness have become widespread as never before—in the popular media, in corporate training programs, and even in hospitals and wellness clinics. Harvard professor Jon Kabat-Zinn describes mindfulness as "paying attention in a particular way: on purpose, in the present moment, and non-judgmentally." Its many benefits include the alleviation of anxiety and depression, lowered levels of stress, as well as overall physical well-being.[14]

Proper training is important. Just today, as we were rewriting this chapter, we came across research published in a current scientific journal suggesting that mindfulness meditation can carry a certain risk of compromising the accuracy of memory. A flawed study, in our humble opinion; we won't go into the whys and wherefores here. Suffice it to say that there can be "too much of a good thing." But one thing is sure: when some scientists start warning people about the potential dangers of a practice that other scientists praise for its health benefits, you know it's an idea whose time has come.

Today's popular mindfulness techniques are many and varied, and they in turn differ from a number of other forms of meditation. Each type has its advantages. All foster a sense of inner calm and promote physical health as well as mental clarity. Some are derived from particular cultural frames of reference or spiritual traditions; some can be seen as culturally neutral and based simply on the mechanics of the mind. We've selected a few representative samples here that are both accessible to beginners and powerful enough to benefit those with some experience who desire to reestablish or advance a practice they've pursued in the past.

Ultimately, we feel that meditation techniques are best considered temporary stepping-stones to a consistent, ever-expanding state of awareness and cognitive acuity. Our hope, and our intention, is that we should be awake and alert all the time, not just during or immediately after these ten- or twenty-minute exercises. One of the great sages of our tradition said something similar with regard to prayer (a very specialized form of meditation): "Would that a person could be praying all day!" But we have to begin somewhere.

We'll start with three simple yet powerful meditation practices. Practice 1 focuses on the way the mind pays attention to the physical body; Practice 2 leverages the relationship between the mind and our emotional state; and Practice 3 works to refine the mind as it receives conscious thought from beyond consciousness, from our inner source of thought.

Any of these techniques will greatly benefit those who use them regularly. The cultivation of consciousness accomplishes far more than merely calming the nerves and improving mental capacity—as we will see when we turn our attention in later chapters to other aspects of internal and outer-directed excellence.

Third-Actors have more opportunity and more motivation than ever to put these practices to good use. If not now, when?

There are numerous variations on Practice 1, including more complicated methods that encourage inhaling, holding the breath, and exhaling to a specific rhythm, and other styles that simply follow the breath without counting. This one is simple and, in our opinion, ideal for beginners. Once learned, attention to the breath can also be applied in quick, abbreviated ways that take only a few moments (see the one-minute meditation sidebar in chapter 3). Note that in many traditions, the breath represents the relationship between the body and the soul.

MEDITATION PRACTICE 1:
ATTENDING TO THE BREATH

Sit comfortably, neither slouching nor rigidly upright, with your shoulders relaxed and your stomach soft and easy.

Close your eyes, breathe through your nose, and notice your breathing as it enters and exits. Is your breath shallow, filling only the upper lungs, or does it penetrate more deeply, toward your abdomen? Don't force it, but as you inhale, visualize the breath descending all the way to the area two or three inches below your navel.

As you exhale, imagine the breath emerging from that same place and traveling up and out back through the nose.

When this process becomes comfortable, silently begin to count the breaths: inhale, exhale—one. Inhale, exhale—two. Inhale, exhale—three. And so on. When you get to ten, start again with one. One to ten, one to ten.

That's it; just pay attention to your breathing by counting your breaths. If you get distracted or lose the count, don't worry about it; just begin again. If extraneous thoughts come along (they will!), just turn your attention back to the breath.

We recommend starting out with a five-minute commitment to this exercise. You could set a timer or keep a watch or clock nearby and gently, slightly, open your eyes to check the time. You might eventually practice this for up to twenty minutes at a time, but even a few minutes makes a big difference. When time's up, take one more full breath, open the eyes, stretch a bit, notice how deeply relaxed and clear-headed you feel, and enjoy the day.

Moving on from being mindful of the purely physical sensation of the breath, let's look at a different meditation style—one that more explicitly engages the heart.

With this technique, pleasant, resonant imagery entertained in our visual imagination evokes positive, nourishing emotions. Of course, when it comes to imagery, there are different strokes for different folks. Some people appreciate the guidance of a meditation coach, while others prefer, once trained in the basics, to explore these techniques at their own pace. Here, for starters, is a sample meditation that has proven popular among many of our students and

MEDITATION PRACTICE 2: RAINBOW VISUALIZATION

Sit comfortably with your hands in your lap and with your feet uncrossed and grounded on the floor. Close your eyes and check in with your breath. Breathe in easily and exhale deeply. Repeat this a few times as you allow the troubles of the past and anxieties about the future to fade away.

Allow yourself to focus on your feet; release any tension or tightness you may feel in your feet. Relax your shins, your knees, your thighs, as you continue breathing calmly and easily while scanning the body and releasing tension as you go. Relax the trunk of your body, your internal organs, your stomach, your lungs, your heart. Relax your shoulders and upper arms. Let all the tension flow from your forearms and your hands and fingers, to a space in the air beyond you, where it will disperse and disappear. Relax your neck; if there's tension there, allow your head to rotate in a slow, spontaneous movement. Relax your mouth and your facial muscles. You are now relaxed from your toes to the tip of your head.

Now imagine yourself floating slowly upward, rising up through the colors of the rainbow. At first you are floating through the red of the rainbow, slowly, effortlessly. Everything around you is red. It fills you with energy and enthusiasm and the desire to act. But you continue to float ... up through the orange ... warm and welcoming ... and you float slowly and gracefully through the intimate orange until you reach the yellow, the color of the sun. It is a happy, balanced color.

Then up, up beyond the yellow to the green, lush and healing, representing fresh starts and rebirth. You feel renewed as you float easily up through the verdant green of the rainbow until you are gliding through the blue, the infinite blue of the sky. It seems to go on forever—and so can you, in a heavenly, weightless frame of mind. Now more soul than body, you enter the mystical purple of the rainbow. It is the color of robes of royalty, of unknown secrets. The purple invites you to leave behind the weighty reality of the physical world as you continue to float.

Now allow all the colors of the rainbow to spin together gracefully in your mind's eye. No one color is greater than any other, as they blend harmoniously to merge into a pure white light. It is the light of kindness and wisdom. Let it rest on your head and shoulders. Feel comfortable basking in its presence. Allow this light of kindness and absolute wisdom to be your constant companion and your friend. You can take it with you wherever you go, and use it to see through the challenges of life more clearly.

When you are ready, allowing that pure white light to remain with you, streaming in front of your eyes, slowly open your eyes.

clients. It begins with a few minutes of progressive relaxation—a means of releasing physical tension in the body that is valuable in and of itself—and then segues to an uplifting visual experience in the eye of the mind.

The third form of meditation we'd like to introduce is somewhat more abstract, as it is simply about allowing the mind to quiet itself, independent of any particular content. It utilizes the natural dynamics of the way thinking navigates the stream of thought that flows into and through the mind. By experiencing a thought at progressively subtler levels of consciousness, we become more attuned to the deep internal source of thought.

In certain traditional cultures, such techniques use specific words or sounds, often called *mantras*. More recently, the method has been adapted to a culturally neutral practice that anyone can use to great advantage, regardless of differing languages or beliefs. One such approach was developed by Harvard professor Dr. Herbert Benson, and presented in his best-selling book *The Relaxation Response*.[15] Meditation Practice 3 is a simplified version that captures the essence of this amazingly effective exercise.

One objective of this mode of meditation is to make a more conscious connection between the words we use (whether in speech or in thought) and the still, small voice of the soul. Words are powerful. The ability to use language to think creatively and communicate effectively is perhaps the most significant faculty that distinguishes humankind from other sentient beings. By connecting these abilities to their source deep within the mind, this practice can enrich

MEDITATION PRACTICE 3:
FLOATING UPSTREAM

This meditation calls for you to prepare by selecting a simple, pleasing word that feels comfortable to say. (Many people do well choosing the word "one.") We are not going to analyze or contemplate the meaning of the word; we're simply going to let it reverberate for a while, and use it as a vehicle to bring our attention to deeper regions of the mind.

Sit comfortably in a quiet place and close the eyes. Take a few breaths and allow the mind to settle for perhaps thirty seconds. Then gently say the chosen word to yourself. Repeat it a few times, and then whisper it to yourself a few times, more quietly each time. Now repeat it mentally, without moving the lips, and allow the word to keep on repeating in your mind, while you simply pay attention to the sound of the word. After a few minutes, you might find that the word will spontaneously change, speed up or slow down, or fall into rhythmic step with your heartbeat or breath. It may even become so quiet and subtle that it is more of an indistinct impulse than an actual word. Or it may not. Whatever happens, just take it as it comes. There's no right or wrong way to do this, as long as it's easy to do. When you find yourself distracted by extraneous thoughts, simply notice that the distraction has happened and turn your attention back to the word.

Here too, as in Meditation Practice 1, you can use a timer (preferably one with a soft, gentle tone) or simply take a peek at a nearby clock or watch. We've found twenty minutes to be an ideal span of time for this meditation. When it's time to stop, take a few deep breaths, stretch, and slowly ease back into the day's activities.

that power immeasurably and actualize our unbounded positive potential. We can bring the peaceful clarity of the upstream source of consciousness to the raging waters of our downstream lives.

In ways that will become abundantly clear in the next chapter, these practices can also help to broaden perspective and develop emotional intelligence. Meditation creates deep relaxation and releases stress, helping us to become more patient, less judgmental, and better able to appreciate other points of view. Embodying this equanimity, we become an inspiration to others, a calming influence amidst the turbulence of life in this diverse world.

Imagine how many problems and conflicts would be readily resolved if we could tolerate and respect our differences, rather than insisting that others must see things our way.

We'll conclude this chapter with a parable from a Jain legend. You may have encountered this story in some form elsewhere; we hope that in the context of these exercises in expanding and deepening our consciousness it will offer new meaning.

THE ELEPHANT PARABLE

Once there were six blind men who lived in a small village. One day, amidst great excitement, the villagers told them, "There is an elephant in our village today!"

As they had no idea what an elephant was, the six blind men decided to go to the center of town to touch the elephant, even though they could not see it. Each of them touched a different part of the huge creature.

"Aha! The elephant is a pillar," said the first man, who had touched his leg.

"No, you are wrong! It is a rope," said the second man, who had touched the tail.

"No, not a rope! It is like the trunk of a tree," said the third man, who had touched the trunk of the elephant.

"It is like a fan," said the fourth, who had touched the elephant's ear.

"It is like a wall," said the fifth, who had touched the elephant's belly.

"It is like a spear," said the sixth, who had touched the elephant's tusk.

They began to argue, each one insisting that he was right. As the argument grew more intense, a wise man happened by.

"What is the problem, my good fellows?" the wise man asked.

"We cannot agree on the nature of this elephant," they replied, and each one shared his perception.

"Ah, but you are all correct," the wise man explained. "Each of you is telling it differently, because each one of you touched a different part. In truth, the elephant has all the features you described."

And so the argument was peacefully resolved, because each man felt validated, and each one understood.

6

Emotional Intelligence

Most folks are as happy as they make up their minds to be.
—ABRAHAM LINCOLN

How often does it happen that you're sure you know the right thing to do but can't get yourself to do it? Or you're well aware that a feeling you're seized with is unreasonable, but can't seem to find your way out of the emotional cul-de-sac you find yourself in?

Or (and this is a subtler, but no less common scenario) you *think* you've straightened out your feelings about someone or something that was bugging you, but when push comes to shove, you're back reacting in the same childish way you thought you'd outgrown?

None of us is perfect. Expecting to be perfect can be a trap that keeps us from getting better a step at a time. So can comparing oneself to others. We may have come to the intellectual realization that we don't need to be better than anyone else, just better than we were yesterday; but then a moment of pressure or stress arrives, and that toxic competitive urge returns. We may have worked long and hard on cultivating the art of empathy, only to discover that we've become so wrapped up in others' emotions we've lost touch with our own.

Yes, we've learned ways of working down dysfunctional feelings and letting them go. Perhaps we succeed more often than not. But you'd think after sixty-plus years of good intentions and working on ourselves we'd finally get it right the first time!

"The longest journey," says Bill W., author of the *Big Book of Alcoholics Anonymous*, "is between the mind and the heart."[16] We'd add that the journey goes both ways, and we make that round trip many times every day.

Each step we take is an opportunity to develop a deeper understanding of emotional intelligence and put that wisdom to work. A heart and a mind that nourish each other, that embrace and allow each other to flourish, become an integrated "heartmind" that can transform conflict into harmony, internally and externally. This may or may not be an explicit part of your mission statement, but whatever your sense of purpose in life may be, this integration can help ensure that you'll fulfill it with grace.

Your Emotional Quotient (EQ)

Emotional intelligence enables us, first of all, to be more consistently aware of moods, feelings, and emotions—our own as well as those of people around us. Moreover, it helps us to understand the processes and perspectives that give rise to those emotional states, and then in turn empowers us to use this information to guide our behavior and inter-actions with others.

The classical standardized IQ test (a quantitative gauge of a person's "intelligence quotient") only measures intel-lectual capacity.

The EQ has recently become an accepted yardstick of emotional intelligence. According to Daniel Goleman, a Harvard-trained psychologist and science journalist who in 1995 authored the definitive, best-selling book *Emotional Intelligence*, non-cognitive skills can matter at least as much as IQ. In fact, Goleman contends, EQ is often a greater indicator of personal effectiveness and success than IQ. Among the principal elements of emotional intelligence, *self-control*, *enthusiasm*, *persistence*, and *motivation* make the difference between merely having good intentions and the ability to take effective action. And *empathy*, another key aspect of EQ, fosters successful relationships.[17]

Our power of empathy tends to be far greater in our advancing years. As a result we can become more adept at true communication on both the giving and receiving ends. This enhanced ability can be attributed to the additional years of interpersonal relationships we have under our belts, or to the fact that having retired from nine-to-five worlds, we can begin to be more selective about those with whom we choose to interact. But the most significant factor lead-ing to deeper empathy may well be our increasing afflu-ence of time. We now have greater ability to slow down, pay attention, listen to what others have to say, and equally importantly, sensitize ourselves to what they're *not* saying.

Let's break this down a bit and take a look at how the elements of EQ unfold in our experience and how the skillful cultivation of emotional intelligence can enhance our performance in the roles we assume in the Third Acts of our lives. The process of achieving emotional resonance in our minds, and cognitive clarity in our hearts, can be seen in four phases:

- **Perceiving emotions.** This is the ability to interpret nonverbal signals, such as body language and facial expressions. Why does that guy seem to be scowling so much of the time? Why are that woman's arms folded so tightly across her abdomen? Your accurate interpretation of such signals can guide you to feel empathy and say the right thing, or at least to avoid saying something insensitive. It can be equally important to notice your own habitual or unconscious body language. The mind can deceive itself, but the body is less likely to lie.

- **Reasoning with emotions.** Rational thinking has the distinct advantage of making room for opposing points of view. Emotions, not so much. Feelings, like love or fear or anger or gratitude, tend to rule the roost and resist change or nuance, often to our detriment. However, emotions have the advantage in passion and power. Emotions also help us prioritize. When we feel passionate about something, that's a pretty trustworthy tip-off that it's not just another item in a laundry list of possible ideas. We need to pay attention to it and unleash its energy. The key to harmonizing intellect and emotion is to leverage the advantages of each and let them listen to each other. Because as we grow older we are generally less anxious about the urgency of everyday life, we have a greater ability to allow the heart to appreciate the mind's perspective. And vice versa.

∾ **Understanding emotions.** Individuals with high EQ, who have developed a rich skill set of emotional and cognitive integration through the years, display greater confidence and trust in themselves, and deeper understanding of others. They also gain a sharper ability to discern appropriate points of intervention in those inevitable situations where minds get stuck or emotions run amok. They will therefore create healthier relationships, achieve more, experience more love and joy, and become adept at helping people get over themselves and get along. It's a talent that, if we feed it and exercise it, just keeps growing!

∾ **Regulating emotions.** The heart, it's often been observed, has a mind of its own. Or rather it has the knack of generating some sort of cognitive activity that looks like thinking but really isn't. The thoughts that usually arise in response to emotion hardly represent our clearest thinking; more likely they are the result not of actual emotion but of the habitual, visceral attitudes and moods that run in the background, waiting for an opportunity to drag us down. A healthy, mature mind rules the heart, albeit with compassion and empathy; it is always ready to validate the heart's true desire. Such a heart, opened and humbled and appropriately empowered, will in turn enrich the mind. Whether young or old, we all have moments when this ideal scenario seems a far cry from our inner reality. But we are neither stuck nor doomed. We have the capacity to become enlightened and enlivened. The secret, as you will soon see, lies in what we call *wait training.*

HOLD THAT MARSHMALLOW!

Goleman cited a well-known study of human behavior performed in the 1960s at a preschool on the campus of Stanford University.[18] A group of four-year-olds was given the challenge of restraining themselves for fifteen minutes from eating a marshmallow placed in front of them. The reward they were offered was a whole package of marshmallows! As the observers watched from behind a one-way mirror, some of the kids were able to wait, while others impulsively popped the marshmallows in their mouths. A middle group engaged in all kinds of antics so they wouldn't succumb to the temptation.

Fourteen years later, this longitudinal study tracked down these children as teenagers. The results were astounding. Those who had resisted temptation at four were now more socially competent, more self-assertive, and better able to cope with the challenges of life. They were more successful across the board, from social interactions to SAT scores, from staying on a diet to pursuing a medical degree. This self-imposed, self-regulating ability to delay gratification for a longer-term goal was a more accurate indicator of success than their IQs or their parents' economic bracket.

The root of the word *emotion* is the Latin *motere*, to move. To exhibit refinement, maturity, and emotional health, we strive to develop the ability to control (or at least moderate or regulate) the volatile movements stirred by our inner feelings. Educators and psychotherapists call it *impulse control*, which, according to Goleman, is the root of all emotional intelligence, since all emotions by their very nature lead to impulses to act.

Like good comedy, impulse control depends on a sense of timing. To a great degree, we regulate ourselves when we are able to consciously enter the gap between thought and action. Between the moment when we become aware of a thought or feeling and the moment when we act on that impulse, there is an opening, an opportunity, a space in which we are free to decide whether to speak or act immediately or to wait until we are more certain as to how we ought to respond. This is called *wait time*—and it makes room for *response ability*.

Let's briefly review the workings of the brain. Our first responder to external stimuli is a lower-order processing center known as the amygdala, or lizard brain (see chapter 5). The amygdala's work occurs quickly: we determine whether a situation is threatening, and if so, the flight-or-fight response kicks in. Then the message is transferred to the limbic system, the seat of our habitual emotions, where the cascade becomes virtually unstoppable. When we respond this way, we are reactive, driven by lower-level thinking.

> *Impulse is the medium of emotion; the seed of all impulse is a feeling bursting to express itself in action. Those who are at the mercy of impulse—who lack self control—suffer a moral deficiency: The ability to control impulse is the base of will and character.*
> —DANIEL GOLEMAN

On the other hand, if we train ourselves to wait when stimuli arrive, we can redirect our thinking to the higher-level center in the cerebral cortex. It's as simple as noticing when a potentially volatile thought or feeling arises and then stepping back and holding on. Take a deep breath or three. Pause; think "calm." We can move from habitual, reactive behavior to creative, conscious *response ability* that is characterized by clear thinking and real freedom of choice. We've all seen toddlers in the throes of the "terrible twos." Some of us were susceptible to similar tantrums (cleverly disguised, of course) well into our twenties and beyond. We don't want to be acting like eight-year-olds in our eighties.

Wait Training

The creative choices we make in those freed moments of wait time have been forged in the crucibles of our lives, composed of the sifted sands of our experience, the product of our spiritual training and core values, our early childhood and higher education, our intellect and intuition, our losses and wins. But they are neither predetermined nor predictable. The better situated we are in the quiet spaces of that gap, the more effectively our collected, selected motivational forces will guide us toward virtue rather than regret.

You can become a thermostat rather than a thermometer, a regulator rather than a simple gauge, aligning yourself intentionally with your value-driven life. A proactive individual sets his gauges for optimal climate control rather than reacting like a thermometer, whose mercury rises and falls with external conditions beyond his control. An emotionally intelligent person is a thermostat, preempting environmental influences, whether they are meteorological, sociological, or psychological. She regulates her thoughts, speech, and deeds with a sense of personal mission, freed from coercion, nourished and empowered by principles.

AFFIRMATIONS: THE SEEDS OF POSITIVITY

Another important component of wait training is building a toolbox of positive thoughts. Psychologists call these positive thoughts *affirmations*. When we introduce these powerful, upbeat aphorisms into the liberated space of our wait time, we neutralize knee-jerk negativity, boost emotional health, and educate the spirit.

Here in the sidebar is a brief selection of some of our favorite affirmations, though you'll probably prefer to come up with your own. With a little effort you can construct a list that's custom-designed to turn around your particular dysfunctional default modes. Some find it helpful to do so in collaboration with a friend or coach who knows them well. To anchor these affirmations in your thoughts, we suggest choosing three or four that really speak to you, then writing them down so you'll have them readily at hand.

To anchor the affirmation still more firmly in your mind, try this: begin several slow deep breaths, and on the third deep inhalation, say to yourself one of the affirmations you find most helpful. Breathe out, inhale again, and silently ponder the next one on your list. Do this from time to time over the course of a few days, and you will blaze a significant trail in your neural pathways: these thoughts will begin to stream effortlessly with your breathing.

Here's another remarkable exercise we use to great effect in coaching workshops. Take a few minutes to write your chosen affirmations with your nondominant hand. That means if you are right-handed, use your left hand, and vice versa. Your "off" hand is more childlike and untrained; it therefore evokes whole-brain concentration. Nondominant writing will help you embed these affirmations more securely and with greater resonance.

With wait training and affirmations in your toolbox, you can begin to examine the particular patterns or triggers

SAMPLE AFFIRMATIONS

This isn't life threatening.

Life gives me exactly what I need and can handle.

People, places, and things don't make me angry (or nervous, afraid, or sad); I make myself that way with my attitude toward them.

On a scale of 1 to 10, how uncomfortable is this?

My value isn't determined by other people's opinions.

My primary goal is peace!

Spirituality is the ability to handle discomfort with dignity.

Calm generates calm.

Calm is strength.

I am solution-oriented, not emotion-oriented.

Perfection is a hope, a dream, and an illusion!

Everyone makes mistakes. That's why pencils have erasers and computers have delete keys.

I am lovable and capable.

The only person I can control or change is me!

that disrupt your emotional equilibrium. These are among the most prevalent ones:

- ∾ Loss of control ("Life would be so much better if the world would just listen to me").
- ∾ Loss of comfort, whether financial or physical.
- ∾ Loss of communication (Simcha struggles with this one; he thrives on verbal interaction).

ᴄᴠ Loss of cooperation ("Why is it so hard for the whole family to be on time for a simple Sunday barbecue?").

ᴄᴠ Loss of honor or appreciation (this one drives Frumma to the brink; she's wired like an only child).

Once you've identified a pattern that triggers your emotional reactivity, examine your list of affirmations and find the one that best addresses it. Write it, say it, breathe it. Most of all, remember to *use* it when you need it.

When you feel your adrenaline pumping and your heart begins to race, *wait*. Just hang out for a while in the gap between stimulus and response. Then aim—select the positive thought that will best address this perceived threat—and shoot: introduce the thought in your mind. Let it reverberate and resonate as it soothes the rough edges of negative emotion.

Building Emotional Intelligence

We might imagine that as we mature, our impulse control and overall mastery of emotional intelligence should automatically advance along with us. But we are creatures of habit. Negative, reactive patterns actually create well-worn grooves—dysfunctional neural pathways in our brains.

To continue to grow, we need to be alert and reevaluate our patterns. Through wait training, we can alter those pathways and find new grooves. We mentioned earlier how current brain research shows that about 90 percent of our thoughts are the same as yesterday's. We must consciously reeducate ourselves to change that, to move forward, not backward. None of us wants to morph into a grumpy old man or an ill-tempered battle-ax.

Shawn Achor, cofounder of the Institute for Applied Positive Research, has taught at Harvard and traveled the globe speaking to large corporations about "the happiness advantage." Achor's research shows that people who keep a gratitude notebook experience a heightened sense of well-being and function more efficiently. He also recommends a commitment to ten minutes of meditation, a ten-minute walk, and one act of kindness daily, along with taking note of what he calls a "wonderful moment" that happened that day. He goes so far as to say that physicians who follow this prescription for twenty-one days will be 19 percent more accurate with their diagnoses! We encourage you to watch his TED talks—entertaining and amazing![19] Big business buys into Achor's ideas because they understand how emotional intelligence and enhanced happiness make for a more productive enterprise.

We can build the muscles of emotional intelligence the way a weight lifter sculpts his physique. The bodybuilder gains muscular definition through many reps with small weights; with large weights, he builds muscle mass. With our small waits, and many repetitions over time, we can become emotionally buff. By working up to larger waits—expanding our capacity for wait time through perceiving, understanding, and regulating emotion over more extended periods of time—we can build emotional muscle mass. (It's not all about the body, or even the heart and mind; there are spiritual dividends as well.)

Here are a few sample longer-term practices you may want to adopt or adapt for your own use in the ongoing effort to build emotional intelligence:

- ∾ Receptivity to constructive criticism is a sign of well-developed emotional intelligence. Before responding defensively to a criticism or complaint, count to ten and tell yourself, "This may be exactly what I need to hear." To your critic, simply say, "Thank you."

- ∾ Food can be a major obstacle, or an amazing training ground, in the cultivation of impulse control. Whenever you feel the urge to eat (regardless of whether it's genuine hunger or self-indulgence), try waiting fifteen minutes before eating. If fifteen is too difficult, begin with five. Or make a commitment to only eat sitting, never standing. Or practice chewing a tasty morsel fifty times before swallowing. With some simple foods, such as whole-grain brown rice, you'll discover new worlds of subtle sensorial delight. Another method is to make a point of consistently leaving the last bite of food on your plate.

- ∾ Children, especially adult children, can be our best trainers. Don't be in a rush to explain to your grown child something you think he did wrong and how he might better handle such situations in the future. Wait (weeks or months, if that's what it takes) until a receptive moment arises in which you're likely to be heard.

- ∾ Refrain from going online and browsing the Internet until noon. (OK, 11:00 a.m.)

∾ While waiting in line at a retail store or bank, work on sustaining positive thoughts.

∾ In conversations, develop the self-restraint never to interrupt another person. Cultivate the art of listening. As Stephen Covey teaches, "Seek first to understand, and then to be understood."[20]

- -

WHAT "I" IS

Think you're a good listener? Consider this story, about a boy who comes bounding in from school, full of enthusiasm.

"Mom! Today I learned something really interesting! I is—"

"No, sweetheart," his mother interrupts, "I am."

"Oh, OK, Mom. I am the ninth letter in the alphabet."

- -

A Final Thought

Before moving on, we want to make one final point about emotional intelligence and positive affirmations. We've saved it for last because we want it to echo through the coming chapters.

We've been emphasizing the power of positive thought—how, by introducing and embracing an uplifting, life-affirming idea in times of negative emotion, we can change our mindset and emotional baseline for the better.

Positive thinking can indeed transform a dark mood or painful feelings to an optimistic, cheerful outlook. However, we are not suggesting the *suppression* of negativity or the muffling of troubling thought.

In our private practices we often encounter people struggling to cope with physical or emotional pain. While we offer many effective therapeutic methods and coaching strategies, we've found that a key to getting better is to first *acknowledge* and *accept* the negative. Sometimes that's as simple as allowing ourselves to feel the pain. If we try to bury, mask, or ignore bad feelings or thoughts, they will more than likely fester beneath the surface and come back to bite us. Happiness applied as a superficial veneer will eventually be exposed as illusory. The lasting efficacy of our positive affirmations lies precisely in the way we simultaneously embrace and accept, rather than suppress or deny, the hard reality of what we want to change. Genuine joy often emerges out of the bittersweet experience of looking at life honestly, fearlessly facing the darkness, and discovering within it the brightest of light.

Creative, transformative energy has been described as a rubber band stretched between two extremes—at one end, the current reality that leaves much to be desired, and at the other end, the vision of what we want to see and bring into being. The tension between the two propels us forward. It's a powerful metaphor for our potential for change.

On that note, let's release this rubber band and let it fly as we apply emotional intelligence to the magical task of transforming our attitudes toward the future and the past.

No Worries, No Regrets

Don't worry about the world coming to an end today.
It is already tomorrow in Australia.
—CHARLES M. SCHULZ

In our experience, having met people all over the world as well as in our own clinical and coaching practices, two negative emotions seem to occur disproportionately in the senior population—worry and resentment. Anxiety about what will or will not be reflects a skewed perspective about the future; bearing grudges reveals a pathological relationship with the past.

In chapter 3, we discussed the rather mystical notion that the universe is being created anew in every moment. Deepening our awareness of the present moment is indeed a powerful way of connecting to this essentially timeless dimension of reality. But however successfully we may have come to the liberating realization that *there's no time like the present*, most of us could use some help internalizing the idea in a meaningful and effective way. Here in the real world, especially as we get older and a little less pressed for time, it's too easy to get hung up about the insults and injustices of the past and worried about what's going to happen down the line.

What, Me Worry?

There's a lovely little tree-lined canal near our home where we frequently walk in the early morning hours. It has a fitness trail with exercise stations, the water is clear, and even in the sultry summer humidity the breezes are beautiful. We see ambitious young joggers shiny with sweat, snowy-white long-necked egrets, beautifully plumed mother ducks followed by fuzzy yellow babies, and parades of fifty-plus walkers, many of whom are out early because they can't sleep. Their stories are written in their gaits, their cervical vertebrae, the lines on their faces.

We are far from being mind readers, but we know these people: They worry about the world, about their children, about their health, about their retirement investments. They entertain worst-case scenarios, engage in a lot of negative future tripping, allow their anxieties to overtake them. Yes, in many cases they have valid cause for concern, but too much worry can lead to chronic, debilitating anxiety. Research has shown that anxiety can disturb your sleep, tax your immune system, raise the risk of post-traumatic stress disorder (PTSD) and other mental health issues, and even shorten your life.

On the other hand, there is an upside to worrying, and most chronic worriers therefore have mixed feelings about their worries. "Got to keep it real," we tell ourselves. "I have to be responsible." "Denial doesn't make problems disappear." Fears of financial distress and physical deterioration are a real part of aging. When we have genuine issues to deal with, it makes sense to worry; we need to be ready for anything. If we keep exploring all the angles and going over every potentially disastrous contingency, we might just figure it out and head off a disaster.

It is difficult to let go of worry, because in some sense your worries have been effective. Even if you decide that you simply must stop agonizing, the effort is likely to have the opposite effect. Remember that mind game we used to play as kids, when you'd turn to a friend and say, "Whatever you do, don't smile"? It inevitably brought on huge smiles, sometimes even gales of laughter.

WORRY TIME

So don't try to "just say no." Instead, you might create a space for worrying in your day. Pick a time and a place, preferably the same time and place every day. During the rest of the day, whenever anxieties come to mind, just jot them down and postpone them until it's "worry time." When the time arrives, go over your list of things to worry about. Decide which are real, which are unlikely, and which are utterly imaginary. If it's real, it's most likely solvable. Take some time to brainstorm several solutions to the problem. And when worry time is over, move on.

By allowing yourself to postpone your worrying rather than trying to stop it, you are gaining control over your thoughts. Postponing your worry is effective because you are not suppressing it; you're simply saying, "I am not worrying about this *now*." Over time you will come to be amazed at how much command you actually have over your once-compulsive emotional tone.

In a 2010 study, scientists from Harvard University investigated how mind wandering affects happiness.[21] They created a smartphone app that periodically asked a few thousand participants how happy they were feeling, what were they doing, and whether their thoughts were focused on the current activity or worrying about something else.

The researchers found that people spend almost half of their time thinking about something unconnected to their current task, and that they were less happy during those moments. Moreover, positive thoughts had little effect on their mood, whereas neutral and negative thoughts made them considerably less happy. The research ascertained that a wandering mind affects happiness more than any activity. These results certainly suggest that recurrent worries are detrimental to our state of well-being, overtake our pleasant moments, and rob us of our joy. Further studies at universities in the United Kingdom indicate that multitasking has adverse effects on IQ as well as on brain density in the areas responsible for empathy and emotional control.[22]

LETTING GO TIME

So in addition to establishing a worry time, it'd be a good idea to also avail ourselves of a "letting go time," specifically with regard to anxiety. Here we can adapt and repurpose some of the exercises we've mentioned earlier. Remember that quick breathing release from chapter 3? Take a moment to breathe in deeply. As you exhale, let go of the past and all its troubles. Breathe in again; as you exhale, let go of the future and all its worries. Now breathe in a third time, and while exhaling allow yourself to arrive fully present to this moment in peace. Practice this periodically throughout the day. You can link this technique to transitions, like getting into the car or to starting a new activity, such as sitting at the computer or preparing a meal.

Guided visualization can also be tailored to letting go of anxiety. Imagine your worries like clouds in the sky. Watch them gently pass, and observe as new clouds arrive. The clouds come and go; some of them may look threatening; but they too shall pass, and you are still you. Because you understand the benefits and practice the art of positive thinking, when you see your thoughts turning gray and gloomy, you can gently escort them to a sunnier place.

If you've ever done a simple stretching exercise and felt the sudden release of muscular tension, you know how sweet it can be. We'll have more to say about this sort of stress relief when we discuss various types of exercise in chapter 14. With practice, it can become almost as easy and automatic to let go of stress as it is to become tense in the first place.

The Power of Optimism

Optimism is not simply an inbred attitude that some have and some don't. It's a challenge, a quality of life toward which we can strive, if and when we so choose. Most importantly, it is its own reward. To anticipate the future with trust and joyful anticipation is one of life's great pleasures. To heed our inner herald of doom and gloom is agony. And optimism works: When we think well, things tend to go well.

Successful people are invariably positive people, and were so before the fact, not simply because they succeeded. Whether we ascribe that phenomenon to faith in a Creator, human charisma and ingenuity, or the law of attraction (an idea that has some basis in traditional wisdom, though we feel it's been distorted a bit by some New Age philosophies), it's difficult to deny. It is not by coincidence that the words "In God We Trust" are written on the dollar bill, that universal icon of affluence.

There are many ways to pump up the trust muscle. We can begin to enrich our perspective simply by recognizing the beauty that surrounds us in nature, starting with the way the sun invariably comes up every morning. It is comforting and encouraging to consider the billions of people who have survived and thrived. We can maintain sensitivity toward those who suffer without obscuring the fact that the world is fundamentally good. We can focus our attention on the expansiveness that is inherent in nature as well as in the evolution of the human commonwealth.

There may well have been events in your personal life that have sparked or inflamed your pessimism: the deal that didn't go through, the mortgage that wasn't approved, some troublesome numbers on a blood test, the deadline

SIMCHA LEARNS SOMETHING SLOWLY

Some forty years ago, a close friend of ours who was about to get married had a private consultation with a great sage and spiritual leader. Among the concerns the prospective groom expressed was his anxiety about earning a livelihood. "How do I confidently start a family without a clue how to support them?" he asked. The sage responded, with a smile, "The same God who manages to feed, clothe, and house billions of people can surely make room for a few more."

Upon hearing about this conversation, I was perturbed. Despite my deep respect for the sage, I could not easily reconcile his answer with my awareness of the starving multitudes around the world. This conundrum stuck with me. Over the course of many years, I would frequently revisit it.

My default mode as a young man was a sense of scarcity, of expecting loss. It took decades of study, introspection, and trial and error to alter my perspective and appreciate the fact that the dominant energy in the universe is benevolent and unbounded. By the time I was pushing fifty, the sage's answer to my friend had begun to make sense—not as denial of those in need, but as profound trust in the source of blessing.

you missed that proved devastating, and so on. But those events are over—or may as well be. What matters is, how do you view your life now? A mixed bag, perhaps, but can you see the bright side? At the very least, somehow you were lucky enough to buy or borrow this book.

POSITIVE AFFIRMATIONS

As we've seen, affirmations can stem the tide of negative thoughts. We needn't resign ourselves to being creatures of habit. Perhaps we really *can* teach old dogs new tricks, even (or especially!) at that most subtle level—thought. It's all about perspective, and a positive perspective can be fed. We have seen the astonishing success of Twelve-Step programs in myriad cases of habitual, addictive, and destructive behavior, turning people back from the abyss and miraculously transforming attitudes. It has worked with people of all religions and no religion, with people from all walks of life.

Affirmations figure prominently in Twelve-Step programs. One key to their success is the initial step of turning problems over to a Higher Power. It is empowering to think that even in the worst of times, there is an intelligent, all-knowing life force involved in the details of our lives, responding positively to our acts of self-control or kindness.

Over the years, we have come to trust in a Creator who has our best interests at heart. This may be an uncomfortable leap of faith for some. But perhaps we can all relate to the notion that each of us has a higher self within; our better angels, if you will; a spark of a soul that represents the best of us. With that core truth in mind, here are a few effective affirmations that nourish optimism and trust:

- I am not my body, my baggage, or my reputation. I am, in essence, as whole and perfect as I was created.
- I am valued and unique. I have my own journey and special mission in this world.

- I accept my feelings.
- I think I can!
- I belong!
- Pain is not a sign of failure. The greatest people in history experienced personal pain.
- Every step forward is a victory; so is every smile, every positive act or thought.
- It is all happening according to a compassionate Master Plan.

Reread these affirmations frequently. Choose a few and post them in conspicuous places, perhaps in ones that may particularly benefit from a positive boost, such as your wallet, your mirror, or the refrigerator. Or select one or two and write them down every day for a week. You always have the power to choose your thoughts. Choose thoughts that make you feel happier and more confident, that help you face your challenges with trust and strength.

Forgiveness: Transcending Blame and Shame

We've all encountered people whose actions have irritated, frustrated, or enraged us. Although those events may have long receded into the past, we still seethe—to our own detriment. It's been said that holding on to anger is like drinking poison and expecting the other guy to die.

In the worlds of medicine and mental and emotional health, forgiveness has become a widespread topic of discussion. Fred Luskin, PhD, is the director of the Stanford

University Forgiveness Project and author of the book *Forgive for Good*.[23] According to his findings, forgiveness can improve mental as well as physical well-being. Forgiveness leads to a reduction of the negative effects of stress and fewer health problems overall. Failure to forgive, on the other hand, may be a more significant risk factor for heart disease than overt hostility. People who chronically blame others for their troubles have higher incidences of such illnesses as cardiovascular disease and cancer. Dr. Luskin found that even *imagining* holding a grudge produces negative changes in blood pressure, muscle tension, and immune response, while *imagining* forgiving someone who has hurt you results in immediate improvement in these same signs.

According to Dr. Luskin, one who practices the art of forgiveness becomes "a hero instead of a victim. Forgiveness helps you get control over your feelings. Forgiveness is a choice. Forgiveness is a teachable skill, like learning to throw a baseball. Everyone can learn to forgive."

Yet forgiveness is not the same as forgetting, ignoring, or condoning bad behavior. It does not necessarily entail reconciling with the offending party; nor does it demand abandoning one's feelings. In other words, learning how to forgive does not change the fact that the people we forgive remain accountable for their misdeeds.

FORGIVING OTHERS

Taking a page from the ethical teachings of an earlier age, contemporary psychology and the self-help literature it inspires have suggested that a perceived offense may actually be seen as a favor. The best way to respond to a seemingly unforgivable wrong may well be to reframe it as an opportunity, a lesson you need to learn, something your soul needs in order to reach its full potential. Your adversary may be holding up a mirror to your own weakness or showing you a path to greater inner strength. We can overcome our grievances by understanding that everything that happens to us is for the good.

In the words of the famous Austrian post-Holocaust psychiatrist Viktor Frankl, "Everything can be taken from a man but one thing: the last of the human freedoms—to choose one's attitude in any given set of circumstances, to choose one's own way."[24] Our choices can be rooted in either a positive or a negative perspective. They can be based on an attitude that sees the universe as random, capricious, or despotic; or we can choose to envision and appreciate the Source of life as loving, generous, and benevolent, and that we are loved, collectively and individually, each of us cherished as an only child.

Does the evidence seem to belie this positive point of view? Change your interpretation of the evidence by exercising your own benevolence. Create new evidence. Overcome the momentum, and change direction with an intentional (not random!) act of kindness. Free yourself from the attachments of the past. Cast a new stone and watch for its ripples in the ocean of existence.

Why would a healthy person give over his attention and his waking thoughts to someone who has done him harm? Why rent space in our consciousness to someone who has

slandered or insulted us? The inevitable consequences of
their offenses are not in our purview. Their rectification is
not our job.

Colin C. Tipping, author of *Radical Forgiveness*, suggests an effective technique for letting go of the offenses
of the past. Write a release letter that proclaims to your
Higher Self that you give full permission for all aspects
of resentment to be lovingly released: "I do hereby forgive
_____. I release him to his highest good, and
set him free. I bless him for having been willing to be my
teacher."[25]

FORGIVING YOURSELF

Such methods can also serve as instruments of self-
forgiveness, for they help us recognize and re-frame our
own negative traits and behaviors as opportunities to learn
and grow. It is constructive to look back and learn from our
mistakes; it's wise to take precautions and avoid repeating
our errors in the future. But for some of us, forgiving ourselves is even more difficult than forgiving others. When we
review the past, we may be filled with paralyzing shame or
remorse. Often the desire to change immobilizes us more
than it motivates us, as we stay stuck with the indignity
of our past misdeeds and allow them to limit our futures.
Remember Tarzan from chapter 1? He would never have
reached his destination and rescued Jane if he hadn't let
go of the last vine before grabbing the one up ahead. How
long must we hold on to blame and shame? Jane is waiting!

The inner critic distorts our perspective. While things are going well, calm prevails. But make a mistake—perhaps something as simple as arriving late for an appointment or forgetting an essential item on a to-do list—and alarms go off, sending danger signals racing to our brain, triggering a flight-or-fight adrenaline rush. Suddenly all our blunders and personal failures flash before our eyes as though underlined with a bright yellow highlighter.

We need to take conscious steps to counteract this syndrome. If we can highlight our wins instead of our losses, we can develop the neural pathways of good memory—the revamped habit of remembering the good.

Your Daily VeGGGies

At this point we'd encourage you to add a vital ingredient to the daily gratitude journal we've been recommending (see chapter 2). For this idea, we are indebted to our friend Miriam Adahan, a respected author and therapist.[26]

In addition to writing down a few things you are grateful for, add one act of personal victory that is worthy of celebration. It takes a minute. The victory doesn't have to be huge. It could be resisting an extra slice of key lime pie, pushing yourself out the door for a ten-minute walk, or calling a friend whom you know needs a bit of consolation or even just a "Hi, what's up?"

If it seems that human nature requires us to remember the things we haven't done or shouldn't have done, with a little effort we can change our nature. We can acquire the habit of endorsing ourselves for small daily accomplishments that afford us value in our own eyes. The positive self-esteem that ensues is not egotism or conceit; it is a force that empowers us to do more good and attain greater heights tomorrow. If you like cute acronyms, you can call this form of journaling your "Daily VeGGGies"—taking note of one Victory and at least three things for which you are Grateful.

Once your Daily VeGGGies have become a ritual, you can add one more rewarding exercise. Take five minutes to record in your journal something positive that happened today. A friend called with good news; your daughter stopped by with the kids; the spouse brought home something beautiful to enhance the decor; or maybe a few words about the gorgeous weather you may otherwise have taken for granted. It beats remembering the difficulties and disappointments. When we write down the nice moments, they become more real; we focus on, reflect upon, and celebrate the good that had until now gone unnoticed.

With conscious effort we can succeed in changing the default ratio of our thoughts from negative to positive. While these methods do not necessarily address habitual patterns of shame and blame head-on, they subtly and indirectly deepen our capacity for forgiveness of others and ourselves.

While we are cultivating new daily routines, here is one last simple yet profound suggestion, which has been researched and acclaimed as effective by leading scientists and experts in positive psychology. It is rooted in ancient rites of prayer: Each night, before you go to sleep, quietly, firmly, and sincerely forgive anyone who has hurt you, wronged you financially, or besmirched your honor. Then dig a little deeper and forgive yourself.

You and I can readily adopt any or all of these processes and add them to our already accelerating state of well-being. By learning to free ourselves from the bondage of future fears and past recriminations, little by little, moment by moment, we bring the quality of timelessness into our relationship with time, including the present time, the *now* in which we live.

This timeless quality does not mean denying the pain of the past or suppressing genuine concerns about the future. Paradoxically, being more present in the moment allows us to become more, not less, attuned to our history and destiny—because both the past and the future are embodied in, *contained within*, the now. In being more fully present, we are actually gaining the ability to heal the wounds and dispel the worries brought on by all that has been or may someday be. It is almost as though by entering the stillness of a singular point in time, we can travel back and forth in time.

Having become more forgiving and less anxious, we are less judgmental, more trusting, and free to exercise greater generosity of spirit in all our relationships and roles. The positive impact upon those we love and inspire is immeasurable.

We'll soon see how the release from worry and regret and the act of forgiving are perfect preparation for the next and final chapter of Part Two: the character development phase of this riveting, fascinating, crowd-pleasing, and deeply gratifying Third Act of our lives.

The Power of Words

May you build a ladder to the stars
and climb on every rung;
may you stay forever young.
—BOB DYLAN

As human beings, our ability to speak distinguishes us from all other creatures. Beasts, it's true, can make their needs and feelings known, but only roughly. Language is our domain and ours alone. It allows us to be rational or magical, emotional or cerebral, productive or destructive.

With the power of words at our command, we can master the subtleties of future, past, and present; the complexities of abstract or concrete expression; and the enchantment of metaphor. With the slightest shift of tone or syntax, words can become powerful tools or formidable weapons. They can make or break a commitment, a reputation, a relationship, a partnership, a marriage, or a life.

Frumma once had the privilege of serving as foreperson of a jury in a court of criminal justice. After three days of deliberation, having thoroughly reviewed the evidence and testimony, the jury marched back in to the courtroom. She stood in the jury box and pronounced, "Guilty, your honor." Those three words sent two men to prison for ten years.

Sometimes less is more. If you think those three words were potent, consider the effect of this two-word sentence, which can determine the future of unborn generations: "I do."

At the risk of getting mystical, allow us to point out that according to the traditional spiritual teachings of great civilizations East and West, from the book of Genesis to the Sanskrit Vedas, every facet of the created universe emerges into existence by the power of speech. Even a single sacred utterance can create a world.

The way we speak defines our reality and expresses who we are, or, perhaps more to the point, who we are *becoming*. The content of our words exposes our values and judgment; the quality of our speech reveals our emotions and inner intent. The words we choose to say or not to say are the artifacts and the indices of our social and emotional intelligence. They are the lyrics of our hearts' songs, the poetry of our souls.

Words of praise and solace uplift the lives of others and grant us grace in others' eyes. As for "sticks and stones may break my bones, but names can never harm me," well, whoever invented that schoolyard taunt didn't know diddly-squat about bullying and invalidating, about the bitter roots of negativity, marital disharmony, and toxic parenting. Criticism, even in jest, can tear a sensitive or wounded person apart.

We'd like to share with you a few practical tips, gleaned from our workshops and coaching tools, about how we can enrich our voices and choices of words. But before getting to the how-to stuff, which tends to sound a little preachy on the page, let's first step back and have a look, as we often have throughout this book, at *context*: where is our language coming from? What is its intent? How does it interface with our core values, our sense of purpose, our cultivation of spiritual and emotional intelligence?

Words Matter

At a pivotal point in our younger days, we had the good fortune to meet a man who would become a teacher and a friend for some forty years. He passed away not long ago, late in his eighth decade. He'd been known far and wide as an expert educator, but to us he was also the grandfather figure we'd never known. Simcha was moved to write an essay, a humor-driven eulogy of sorts, recounting some of the things he'd learned from the man. Chief among them was this simple truth, spoken in a moment of wistful candor: "The single most significant thing a person can do in this world is to alleviate someone's suffering." Scarcely a day goes by that we don't remember and take to heart that statement.

Words spoken from the heart, it is said, enter the heart. If our hearts and minds are aligned, if our perception is consistent with our innermost intention, if our words hark back to our deepest core values—in other words, if we are *whole*—then our aim will be true and our words will heal.

In our day-to-day existence, whether we're aware of it or not, we're forever telling ourselves stories. The words we use in our internal dialogues mold our perception of reality. When we then give voice to those thoughts, we offer our versions of reality to others, who may or may not be inclined to agree. Is it a good story? Does it uplift us and them? If it's tragic, does it at least imply a potentially redemptive end?

We need to define our terms before presuming to speak; we need to consider another's inner perspective before assuming it'll be heard the way we meant it. Think about how significant words have been in the conflicts and covenants of history—the duels to the death fomented by someone's broken word; the shattered pacts and treaties that underlie clashes of civilizations; the slander, defamation, and libel suits that clog our courts; the escalating insults and accusations that spark and perpetuate political strife. Note the great weight given to vows in the biblical literature and to the importance of honesty and sincerity in our ethical codes. We may not be players on such grand, global scales, but our words are no less powerful to those around us.

Can we be as careful about what comes out of our mouths as we are about what goes in? The mouth is an interface, not just on the way in, from the grocery store to my belly, but on the way out, from my sense of purpose to the outside world. Impulse control and attention to detail are called for in both directions.

Silence Is a Part of Speech

Just as skipping or delaying an occasional meal can help clean up our act in the culinary department, silence is a great tool for rectifying the power of speech. In the past we have experimented with various ways of exercising some verbal restraint—for example, steering clear of any semblance of gossip, even for a short time. Challenging, but it can grow on you. We've tried to avoid complaining between the hours of 6 and 7 p.m. We've instituted weekly roundtable gratitude sessions at family dinners, each person taking a turn to voice appreciation for something that happened during the week. A friend of ours with a less than golden tongue decided he was going to put a dollar in a charity box every time he cursed. Such ruses won't make us perfect, but they'll help us understand and internalize the principle of carefully choosing our words. We have grown to respect the strength, the compassion, and even the efficiency that accrue from guarding one's tongue.

Is your next statement going to spread love and encouragement, or might it be better to choose silence instead? When you open your mouth to speak, will you be releasing positive or negative vibrations into the universe or into your living room? In short, are you a beacon of light or an SOB?

Words are an investment, so spend wisely. Offer your significant other one compliment, one "I love you," and one sincere "thank you" every day. Yes, we understand: some of us are not all that demonstrative by nature. Do it anyway. It's good to acknowledge the kind things your partner

LYING IN WAIT

A mentor of ours told us a story about how, as a teenager, he was a pathological liar, and how he changed. In a notebook small enough that he could carry it around in his shirt pocket, he made a mark for every lie he told in the course of a day. The sum total was fifty lies. He resolved to tell one less lie every day. So the next day, after ticking off forty-nine lies, he was able to restrain himself until the next day, when he told forty-eight lies. The next day he told forty-seven, and so on. Each day it got a little easier to hold himself back. By the time he cut down to about ten lies a day, he had grown so accustomed to telling the truth that he had to force himself to make up a few lies at the end of the day just to fulfill the quota. By the fiftieth day he had become an honest young man.

does, even though it might seem OK to take these deeds for granted after all these years. Especially for those of us who are in second marriages, such verbal appreciation can be a salve to heal old wounds.

One of the more woeful stories we've heard is about a mother who served dog food to her family one evening for dinner. Everyone was shocked. "Well, none of you has ever told me that you enjoy my cooking," she explained. "I figured I might as well take the easy way out."

Enlightened educators impress upon us the importance of emphasizing the positive, and of being *specific* about it.

"You are so kind!" is an encouraging thing to say to a child, but it doesn't compare to "I noticed the kind way you shared your dessert with your baby sister when she was crying at lunch today."

Children are built with words. Addressing a specific action makes it easier for them to internalize the praise, to own it, and embody it. On the other hand, negative outbursts like "you're so lazy . . . messy . . . selfish . . . disorganized . . . inconsiderate . . . fat" are destructive prophecies that can brutalize a self-image more severely than we ever want to know. In this respect, we are all as vulnerable as children.

But enough of admonitions, lest we fall into the very trap we suggest you avoid and overemphasize the negative. We'll just point out a few more toxic no-no's, but place them within the safe boundaries of a sidebar. That way you can feel free to ignore them or revisit them some other time if you've had enough well-meaning advice for now.

. . . .

BEWARE THE TOXIC TONGUE

Avoid emotionally charged phrases like "a killer headache," "she's driving me crazy," or "I'm such a basket case!"

Stop yourself from being a prophet of doom, as in "You think this is bad? Just wait!" Or, "It's getting hard to remember names. I'm probably developing Alzheimer's." Or, "Now that my husband is gone, I'll be lonesome the rest of my life."

Don't talk like a victim. "She made me so angry!" Really? Like you had no choice with your reaction? "I can't get any-

thing done as long as I live in this stupid place" ascribes more power to the place than to you.

Be conscious of limiting language. Don't say, "I can't" when the reality is that you don't want to. Don't say "I don't have the energy" when the truth is you're just not all that excited about doing it.

Temperamental words like "always" and "never" can be dangerous. "You never help me" or "you always show up late" aren't constructive. Sometimes he does help; and she does, in fact, often arrive on time.

. . . .

Can we in fact transform our propensity for discouraging, insecure language into words that will build confidence and trust? Yes, indeed we can.

The Language of Trust

We generally think of language as a tool for communicating with our fellow humans, but it's much more than that.

We've already mentioned the internal dialogue, that sometimes conscious, often under-the-radar mental murmur that continuously describes and defines the way we see the world. In previous chapters we've discussed some ways in which we can apply meditation and affirmations to help us rewrite our inner stories and cultivate self-forgiveness, confidence, and courage. Here too, wise word choices can be just as important when we're speaking to ourselves.

THE ROLE OF PRAYER

Another use of language—often overlooked, if not entirely dismissed, because it is so commonly and so easily mis-understood—is *prayer*. Prayer is not exactly internal, like meditation, though it has an internal, meditative dimension. Nor is it directed toward an "other" in the same way as communication among peers.

According to a recent AARP survey, about 40 percent of today's baby boomers pray daily.[27] They pray with words of gratitude and praise; they pray for the fulfillment of their physical needs. They pray for understanding and insight and clarity. They pray for the recovery of ailing loved ones. They pray for inner calm, and they pray for world peace. They pray for their team to win the championship, or to be blessed with the winning lottery ticket. Some of the 60 percent who don't pray regularly will suddenly turn to prayer in times of trouble, like the proverbial atheist in the foxhole.

To whom do we pray, and with what sort of expectations?

The majority of mankind apparently believes that there is a Source, a Creator, a Higher Power who is accessible, who hears our words, and who cares about what we are say-ing, feeling, and doing. The Gallup organization conducts an annual survey of beliefs. Results vary with the different ways they choose to phrase the questions, but recent polls have indicated that as many as 94 percent of Americans are believers.[28]

We are not interested here in attempting to prove or disprove the existence of a deity or in discussing the benefits and shortcomings of organized religion. We're just citing the fact that most of us ascribe some value to the process of prayer, that is, reaching out to our Higher Power (whatever we may mean by that) with words.

We'd also like to make a deeper point. Though there is value in the simple, humble act of praying for personal needs (and it need not be superficial or selfish), prayer is not only asking for help from above or beyond. Prayer is also a means of self-examination, of fathoming the inner recesses of memory, of catalyzing and inspiring personal change. In our own tradition, the root of the Hebrew verb *l'hitpalel*, *to pray*, also means *to judge oneself.*

Prayer therefore can be a powerful tool to integrate the emotions with the intellect. Has a life experience rendered us sad or mad or traumatized? Verbalizing our feelings can lead to introspection. Enhanced self-awareness can open the conduits to our higher wisdom and empower us to change. A practice of honest self-assessment can help us grow more trustworthy. Turning that feeling outward can help us learn to trust.

And so we simultaneously turn within and look beyond ourselves—not just to address our problems or to identify and satisfy our needs, but to connect with a deeper dimension of the soul.

If prayer is not yet a part of your life, we invite you to set aside a fixed time daily to experiment with the possibility that it works. It might be in a formalized style, through a prayer book or chanting or reciting psalms; or perhaps you'll be more comfortable with spontaneous conversation, using words that resonate for you.

An early morning expression of gratitude for another day to enjoy can chase away the negative thoughts that creep into our subconscious when we sleep. Ending the day with thoughts of forgiveness can send us off to sleep in a loving frame of mind and encourage us to anticipate peace in our homes, our hearts, and our universe. Gratitude and forgiveness are a far cry from bracketing our waking hours with a default vibe of anxiety or resentment or an expectation of the same old mediocrity day after day.

THE FLIP SIDE OF PRAYER

When we turn the conventional notion of prayer inside out, we discover the most potent power of words. It's fine to ask for blessings from above; we are most wholly human, however, when we *offer* blessings from the depth of our own generosity of spirit. In fact, it's the very act of surrendering to a Higher Power that empowers us as agents and channels for the dominant force in the universe—divine benevolence. The blessings we give are the mirror image of the blessings we receive—and vice versa.

So we bless one another with our best wishes for a safe trip, a speedy recovery, or success in an impending adventure.

These are not just empty words. Our spoken blessings are powerful. There is much more clout than we imagine in that automatic "Bless you!" that follows a sneeze, or in those seemingly inane expressions like "Have a great day!" or "Feel better soon!" or even "Happy birthday!" Our blessings embody our heartfelt kindness and compassion; they initiate a vibrational path towards goodness.

Yet we shy away from using the ability to bless with which *we've* been blessed—perhaps because we've been soured by the cool cynicism that pervades the prevailing culture. Or maybe just because we forget how powerful we really are.

Imagine getting a call from a friend or bumping into an acquaintance on the street and instead of engaging in the usual chitchat, being treated to a powerful, magnificent, unsolicited blessing. "May your life be filled with joy and peace! I wish you perfect health and prosperity! And may all your heart's desires for good come true!" How would that feel?

And how would it feel to step out of your routine for a moment to call or email or (even better!) speak face-to-face with a friend or loved one, just to extend your sincerest blessings, out of the blue? Would such an act of kindness become something to be proud of in your day? And how would it feel if you were to establish a personal ritual whereby you did that every day for a week? What kind of a week would that be?

In a world that too often feels harsh and uncaring, your attention to the power of words can make a difference—one day, one relationship, one life at a time.

We have a reason for placing this chapter here at the conclusion of Part Two. Language is the interface between who we are and our interactions with our world. Our words arise out of the deep silence of our essential selves, driven by our sense of purpose, born of our wisdom and understanding, set to the music of our heartfelt emotional lives. There's always a risk involved in our choices of words: How will they be received? Do they line up with our genuine intention? And are we telling the truth, even to ourselves?

In Part Three, we'll apply the strengths we've cultivated thus far in a few key relationship-based, pragmatic aspects of aging well. Let's remember that we need to listen carefully, even as we speak, both with the inner ear of our own true selves and through the ears of our loved ones.

Beautiful young people are accidents of nature.
Beautiful old people are works of art.

—ELEANOR ROOSEVELT

PART THREE

We're well on our way. We've redefined *retirement* as *renewal*.
We have retooled, refocused, and rededicated our lives
to embrace the *now* and create anew.

Our world is made of relationships—the playgrounds and proving
grounds of our lives. Healthy relationships can help make us
whole. But striving to find completion in our relationships with
others can also make us acutely aware of the ways in which
we are not yet whole inside our own skins.

Wholeness is an art form. By the time Act Three rolls around, we
are ready to get it right. First, in our families: as mates or parents,
as caregivers or storytellers, as sages and lovers. Then in the public
sphere: as community leaders, mentors, team builders at home
and abroad. And through it all, as healthy, creative individuals—
balanced, poised, self-contained, charged with both a vigorous
sense of purpose and the patience to let it all unfold.

9

Making Love Last

The best time to plant a tree was twenty years ago.
The second best time is now.

—CHINESE PROVERB

The romantic dream of soul mates who complete each other is one of those archetypal fantasies that never get old. It's why we cry at weddings, and why we dance. It's why we'll risk life and limb in search of true and lasting love. It's why we stick it out through thick and thin in a marriage gone stale . . . or why, sometimes, we don't, and divorce, and then pick ourselves up and try again.

Maybe you're decades deep in a stable relationship. The kids are grown, the mortgage is paid off, and things seem richer in so many ways. You've gained insight and understanding; you've weathered the inevitable doldrums, seen the threatening storm clouds of emotional infidelity drift away. Yes, he still has that annoying habit of checking his phone at the dinner table, but you forgive him. Yes, there's still that thing she does that irritates the hell out of you. But you behave yourself.

Maybe you haven't been so lucky or smart. Mistakes may go uncorrected. Hearts may ache from tragic loss or hope unfulfilled. Yet the dream persists. It is hardwired, built-in, inexorable: Adam and Eve are one, in essence, and each seeks oneness in the other.

We've come to believe that creating and sustaining a good and growthful marriage is the single most important undertaking in our lives. It is certainly the most fruitful one. Marriage is an opportunity for a couple to help each other reclaim wholeness, to heal the inner child, and to experience and express unconditional trust and love. It is our rectification, our prescription for transformation and emotional health.

Yet even the most highly evolved couples have to stretch beyond their respective comfort zones to build a good marriage. It takes sustained, continuous work. At the risk of wielding a well-worn cliché, success in marriage, like success in every other important venture, is the result of 5 percent inspiration and 95 percent perspiration.

OK, fine—so precisely *how* do we make love last? Could it be all about attraction and affinity, the urge to merge? Not likely, once we move past the magnetism or the initial rush and get to know one another for real. Rare indeed is the couple that can keep passionate love fresh and exciting in the face of conflicting perspectives and shifting agendas.

Then is it more about respect? Establishing functional boundaries, acknowledging and accepting differences, making room for the other's otherness?

Of Otherness and Oneness

Whether or not opposites attract (a dicey proposition, we've observed), love and respect are opposites that *interact*. If we stay fluid and flexible, if we are able to balance the romantic and the pragmatic aspects of a relationship, love and respect will mutually and dynamically morph into one another. Marriage isn't about changing or educating your significant other. It's about fostering a relationship based on both respect for our partner's individuality and love of the ego-free magic that happens when we meet. It's also crucial that we understand and remember that love and respect are not simply amorphous emotions that arise out of forces beyond our control. Love and respect are both verbs. They are actions we choose to take, behaviors we cultivate.

The essential first step is to believe and understand that *nothing in the world is more important than establishing and maintaining an emotionally healthy intimate relationship with the other half of your soul.* This begins, perhaps, by simply acknowledging that he or she is indeed the other half of your soul.

The second step is equally imperative: *Take full responsibility for the things you can change in your own attitude and behavior without demanding or expecting change from your spouse.* The tools at our disposal lie in three distinct toolboxes—our thoughts, our speech, and our deeds:

ɷ We can replace divisive or critical *thoughts* about our spouses with positive, endearing thoughts, simply by paying attention to the things we appreciate (see chapter 6).

- ∞ We can *speak* more respectfully, more gently and generously, and listen more empathically (see chapter 8).

- ∞ We can go out of our way to perform *acts* of kindness, without keeping score or expecting anything in return.

Paradoxically, the return on this investment—the fulfillment we experience as a result of such self-sacrifice—knows no bounds. Marriage is the only relationship in which we can achieve and experience oneness in every dimension of our lives—spiritual, intellectual, emotional, and physical. With practice and commitment, we can cultivate a marital bond that says loud and clear: There is no place where "I" end and "you" begin. Even though we are so unlike each other, we surprise and delight each other with our differences at every turn.

What we need to do—what we are finally, uniquely capable of doing—is to bring our vitality, our spirit, and our potency to the space between us and our partners in life. Among other things, that means committing ourselves to uninterrupted quality time together every day, no matter what. If we seal up the emotional energy leaks, we become partners for real.

The Sound of Silence

There is no lack of advice out there (some of it good!) about how to communicate with a spouse. We have plenty to say about this as well, but we'd like first to suggest something you might find counterintuitive: Quality time in a marriage is not necessarily all about effective communication. At its core, it may be more about silence. A couple that is comfortable enough to sit quietly together and simply rest in each other's presence might just have discovered the secret to an unbreakable bond.

Creating a successful marriage begins with what we don't do and don't say. It takes refinement and impulse control, for example, to abstain from making disparaging or sarcastic comments. To refrain from reminding our spouses of what they didn't do, or did wrong, makes room for inner appreciation and builds patience into a relationship. When we're tempted to deliver a message that carries a lot of emotion, it may be time to take a few deep breaths and quiet the mind instead. One of the great wise men of all time, Hillel the Elder, may have had something like this in mind when he turned the Golden Rule around from "Do unto others as you would they would to unto you" to "Don't do unto others what you wouldn't want done unto you."

When we do speak, it's important to be cognizant of our tone of voice and our facial expressions. We need to work on filtering out judgmental or cynical nuances. In those inevitable moments when you do need to bring up a touchy subject, it can be helpful to first consciously relax your face and jaw—maybe even practice it in front of a mirror a few times—to make sure you come across positively. If you anticipate a bit of friction, change confrontation to curiosity. Ask your spouse questions, in a calm, detached tone, about the issue that bothers you. The subtle message is that you are looking for a solution rather than a battle or a victory.

Remember, though, that there can be a fine line between cultivating impulse control and walking on eggshells—and that one of the prime prerequisites to lasting love is *spontaneity*. Having developed the emotional sensitivity it takes to treat your partner with the same respect you would a stranger, you'll feel free to celebrate life together, playfully, without needing to fix each other. To have fun without undue inhibition, caution, or constraint.

RITUALS REVISITED

Positive and purposeful interactions are the vitamins that keep relationships healthy. And just as vitamins are most effective when taken regularly, it's wise to develop rituals to help your relationship flourish.

Rituals, as we discussed in chapter 3, are very precise behaviors, performed at specific times, motivated by deeply held values, and designed to support and reinforce a desired quality of life. Initiating and establishing a ritual can be complicated, but once you're in the groove, maintaining it becomes relatively easy. And it need not be seen as repetitious. Pay attention: there is newness in it. Each small incremental step unleashes a cascade of positive feelings and strengthens your resolve to keep growing—not just in the specific realm of the ritual at hand, but in other areas as well.

If this were a couples workshop or a coaching session, we might stop here and ask you to think about the kind of rituals you'd like to introduce in your marriage—enjoyable, meaningful activities that would make you and your partner happier and improve your marital bond. We'd probably make some specific recommendations based on your unique personalities, interests, and issues. Then we'd advise you to schedule them into your planner. If you feel you can do that now, great—go ahead! Take action. And remember that scheduling them doesn't exempt you from actually doing them. Why risk losing your way along the infamous road that's paved with good intentions?

Languages of Love

Frumma has a client, a stay-at-home mom (not that there's anything wrong with that) whose husband comes home after his tough day at the office at more or less the same time each evening. Frumma advised her to have the phone in her hand when he comes in, pretend to be on a call, and say, "Oh, sorry, I'll have to get off. My husband just arrived, and I really want to spend time with him!" Your soul mate needs continual reassurance that he or she is the most significant human being in your world. She really is, you know. For each of us, such assurance comes in a different form.

We like the guidelines found in Gary Chapman's bestselling book, *The Five Love Languages*. He postulates that your partner has a primary language that you must identify and learn to speak in if you want him or her to feel loved. Here is a quick synopsis of these languages.

- ∾ For some it is *positive affirmations*: words of praise and appreciation.

- ∾ The second language is *acts of service*, for those to whom actions speak louder than words.

- ∾ The third language is *gifts*. They need not be expensive—a small bouquet of flowers, a well-phrased refrigerator magnet—proof that you're thinking of each other when not together.

- ∾ If your partner's love language is *quality time*, giving undivided attention is the best way to show your love. Some guys think they can watch a football game, read an interesting post on Facebook, and listen to their wives all at the same time. That may well be, but it is not speaking the language of quality time. So turn off the TV, put down the smartphone, gaze into your mate's eyes, and listen and interact. "Undivided" is the magic word in this equation.

- ∾ The last of these languages is *physical touch*: hugging, kissing, sexual intimacy, or perhaps simply a massage. If this is your spouse's language, the most meaningful gift comes when you initiate the affection.[29]

Regardless of the particular love language in play, it is important to make eye contact when your mate is speaking. Stop whatever you are doing and listen. Resist the impulse to interrupt. Remember Stephen Covey's maxim, "Seek first to understand, and then to be understood."[30] Learn to

THE LOGISTICS OF LOVE

An extraordinary couple we knew years ago once shared a small, secret agreement they'd made between themselves: never to call out to each other from another room. If one wanted the other's attention, he'd first get up, walk over to where she was, and speak with her face-to-face. Beautiful.

Even knowing this, however, we'd occasionally default to the easy, taken-for-granted habit of yelling from across the house—until we began to see how such subtle turbulence erodes the quality of communication. Think about it. Imagine how deeply loved your partner will feel, knowing you care enough to get up off your own butt and give due respect to his or her personal world!

become an empathetic listener. Paraphrase what your mate is saying in your own words, and then ask, "Did I get you? Have I understood you correctly?"

Life moves swiftly, so we must work hard to create quality time. Daily, weekly, or monthly, on vacation or during staycations, ritualize your time together. Go out for breakfast or lunch, and turn off the phones. Take frequent walks in nature, and turn off the phones. Collaborate to generate a list of things you would like to do together, and then do them. Look at old photos together. Listen to the music your partner loves; explore music that's new to the two of you together. Tell each other your childhood stories—and turn off the @#!$%*# phones!

The Purpose-Driven Relationship

Many two-career couples drift apart because they work in different environments or pursue different sorts of goals. Even after retirement it can take some effort to ensure that your significant other hasn't become more *other* than *significant*. Yet every couple also has shared goals, and these are the pillars upon which their relationship rests. However busy or preoccupied you each may be, make it a point from time to time to rekindle and pursue the interests you have in common, to deepen your understanding of the values you share. It will help you stay focused and passionate together as a couple, and mutually respectful in those areas where your individual interests may not converge.

In the same vein, find the time to get together and make plans—not just about practical to-do lists for the coming week, but also about your long-term dreams and the meaningful steps you can take toward achieving them. That vacation by the seaside cliffs of Maui, that camping trip in the Smoky Mountains with the grandkids, that organic herb and vegetable garden in the backyard—they won't happen by themselves. Nor will your memoirs write themselves or your oral history record itself. Make the space to envision the future together, and to follow through. Keeping your marital *raison d'être* on a front burner and on your active agenda will enrich your marriage immeasurably.

NOURISHING TRUST

Again (we can't emphasize this too much!) marriage thrives when we establish unity on all four human levels: spiritual, intellectual, emotional, and physical. These are not separate compartments of our lives; they are intertwined. Although there's no simplistic formula for cultivating such oneness, we've come to understand that the thread that weaves these four aspects of a relationship together is *trust*. We've seen self-development and relationship workshops that incorporate physical trust-building exercises. Can you remain totally relaxed while letting yourself fall, knowing your partner will catch you? Can you close your eyes and let your spouse lead you through a maze?

The emotional dimension of trust can be more elusive. How do we grow a strong, well-funded emotional bank account?

The need for honesty is, of course, a no-brainer, but certain nuanced forms of dishonesty can easily trip you up. Exaggerating or understating the way you feel, for example, erodes the openness between partners. Saying you like something that you really don't, or insisting that an incident didn't bother you when it really did, will probably lead to further miscommunication, mistaken assumptions, or even recriminations down the line. When we tell small untruths or settle for partial truths, it can become a habit, thus diminishing our credibility in situations where our mate needs to rely on the weight of our words.

By the same token, stay honest, but not tactless. There is no harmless way of saying, "You seem to be gaining weight."

Avoid sarcasm. In our house we say, "Kidding causes tension." Humor is great, but not at the expense of your soul mate, who *also* has a vulnerable inner critic, just as you do. The snarkiness that abounds in today's popular culture is almost as destructive to the institution of marriage as the episodic adventures of glamorous adulterers. Those of us who grew up on *Father Knows Best* and *Ozzie and Harriet* could probably have predicted the endangerment of the American marriage when the new wave of situation comedies hit the airwaves. Highly evolved, loving relationships are built on respect and trust. Sarcasm and cheap shots that lower your spouse's self-image are counterproductive even if they are said in jest.

The inestimable power of words (see chapter 8) is nowhere as potent as it is in marriage. A positive, encouraging word, offered with a smile—even a text message graced with an upbeat emoticon—can be a gift of great value. We firmly believe that many of civilization's greatest contributions to science, literature, and industry were created only because some innovative genius's spouse said something supportive as he or she left home for the office or the lab.

The interest that accrues in a couple's joint emotional bank account will inevitably be reinvested in the intellectual and spiritual dimensions of their relationship. Trust and esteem nourish insight and wisdom. We try to make

FIVE THINGS I LIKE ABOUT YOU

Some couples build confidence by composing hokey little lists of the things they appreciate about each other. Then they'll sit together at the dining room table and take turns reading them out loud. Contrived? Maybe, but we can assure you that most people who try this exercise treasure the recognition and look forward to repeating it. Here's a brief, candid sampler:

1. *I appreciate how polite you were toward my sister last night. Wasn't easy, I'm sure.*

2. *I love that you squeeze the sponge dry after washing a dish.*

3. *Thanks for texting me that you'd be ten minutes late.*

4. *The way you incline your head when you're thinking about something makes me want to climb into your brain.*

5. *When you leave home early and I'm still in bed, I love the sound it makes when you lock the door behind you. I feel protected.*

time to study together and discuss meaningful, sacred texts daily. Even more than the intrinsic value of the learning, there is nothing so delicious as the ongoing dialogue between a husband and wife about the ideas and ideals that matter most to both. These shared excursions of mind and soul also add value to the simple things, to the most menial of tasks. Who could object to ironing a shirt or scrubbing the occasional pot, knowing that doing so will clear the decks and free us up for a few more moments of life's finer pursuits?

Marriages may be made in heaven, but they often find their most genuine expression in the kitchen or the laundry room (not to mention, as we'll soon see in the upcoming chapter, in the bedroom). The little-known secret about the refined heights of spirituality is that it shows its truest, brightest colors in this down-to-earth, hard-to-handle, pain-in-the-neck physical world. Which is, after all is said and done, where marriage happens.

10

Intimacy:
The Inner Sanctum

Those who have never known the deep intimacy
and the intense companionship of mutual love
have missed the best thing life has to give.

—BERTRAND RUSSELL

Every individual is an entire universe, distinct from every other. We may think we understand those closest to us, but can we truly fathom the mysterious depths of anyone's unique inner world?

With selfless love, empathy, and an invitation, we can grow closer. It takes work, but the effort is among the most gratifying endeavors a person can pursue. Its reward is a glimpse into the innermost regions of the human spirit; even more than that, it is a mirror that reflects shining light back upon our own secret soul and connects us, soul to soul.

The word *intimacy* has become a euphemism for physical sex. Such linguistic decorum, of course, is nothing new—take for example today's sly circumlocution, "He *knew* her in the biblical sense," which harks back to Genesis 4:1: "And Adam knew Eve." Too often, however, the euphemism obscures the painful reality that as physical sex has become progressively more commonplace and casual, real intimacy has become more rare.

The Evolution of Romance

At twenty-five, our robust vitality and raging hormones probably lent a different quality to our sex lives than we are likely to experience at sixty-plus. We would venture to say, however, that sex can be *more* pleasurable, and yes, more genuinely intimate, after sixty. First of all, the level of comfort and self-acceptance that comes with maturity renders us more amenable to emotional bonding. We have more compassion and patience. We are better attuned to a partner's nuanced vibes and subtle signals. Just the fact that we are not in a rush can be exquisite, especially if we don't have very specific expectations.

Much is made of the hormonal differences between men and women. Testosterone, we are told, is a Martian substance, and therefore dominates in pushy, militant, controlling males. Estrogen-driven females hail from Venus and tend to be motivated by a kinder, gentler, more beauty-oriented aesthetic. Clichés, of course, but generally not far off the mark—in our younger years. As we age, however, things change.

In peri-menopause, as a woman's reproductive cycle begins to wind down (usually in her forties or fifties), the

HOW OFTEN?

"How often?" is a question (or an issue) in many marriages. The optimal frequency of physical intimacy will vary with both personal preferences and the state of one's health, not to mention with age. Once a week is an oft-cited rule of thumb, either as a minimum or as an average, for those well past the age of peak performance. But rules, as they say, are made to be broken—in this case, in either direction, depending on the situation. There are myriad health benefits associated with sexual relations, including stress reduction, natural anti-depressant effect, and a boost to the immune system. As a preventative measure, physical intimacy can reduce risks of breast and prostate cancers, heart attacks, and strokes. For increasing the elasticity and the appearance of the skin, it's better than Botox. Sexual activity can even help lower blood pressure for some, and it produces the hormone oxytocin, which in turn stimulates emotional bonding and generosity of spirit.[31] On the other hand, excess can exhaust a person and drain vitality. Especially for people who are frail or in a depleted condition, more moderation is warranted. A trusted health care professional can help determine an appropriate, balanced approach. And frank discussion between partners helps us see eye to eye.

body produces declining amounts of estrogen. Similarly, around his mid-forties a man's production of testosterone begins to diminish, though normally at a much slower pace. The more obvious manifestations of these changes are lowered libido in both genders, dryness and reduced elasticity in women's reproductive organs, and perhaps erectile dysfunction and/or loss of muscle mass in men. On the physical level many people find it difficult to adapt to such shifts, and they experience varying levels of disappointment or frustration. Therapeutic strategies can range from pharmaceutical solutions, which may or not prove effective and often involve side effects, to more natural, holistic approaches and behavioral adjustments. We've seen, however, that as with many other types of health challenges, if we can gain a deeper understanding of the emotional and spiritual dimensions of what seems to be a problem, we might just discover that the silver lining can disperse the cloud.

It turns out Mars and Venus are not as far apart metaphorically as they are in space. In fact, their orbits eventually intersect. With the maturity and hormonal realignment that accompanies age, we're not so polarized as we once were. As men become less driven by testosterone and discover their inner estrogen, they tend to become softer and more (dare we say it?) civilized. (Surely you've noticed how much sweeter Grandpa can be than Dad.) And women often gain an assertive, self-confident demeanor, less susceptible to tidal waves of emotion (to whatever extent those stereotypes are real). This information can prove invaluable not just in family meetings and decision-making conclaves, but in the bedroom as well.

An influential relationships counselor we know became successful and effective expounding on his own proprietary stereotypes, most of which rang true. He'd say, for example, that by and large men want to be respected and women want to be appreciated. A master of discretion and modesty, he would encourage couples to discover their own ways of translating that suggestion into mutually satisfying behavior in the realm of eros and sexual intimacy.

It's been our observation that in the Third Act, roles and expectations shift, sometimes subtly and sometimes dramatically. Older men may desire to be more cherished than respected, and mature women have learned how to command an ever-deepening measure of respect. Moreover, though conventional wisdom suggests that emotional intimacy is more challenging for men than for women, we've seen that the reverse may just as frequently be true, especially with advancing age.

The interplay between emotional bonding, physical affection, and the sharing of meaningful ideas creates a triple-braided tapestry that is not easily unraveled. Intellect is as important an erogenous zone as the skin and flesh. Both provide pathways to our hearts; conversely, the blossoming of emotional satisfaction opens both our minds and our readiness to touch and be touched. Naturally, people with long life experience have gathered myriad tips and tricks over the years that—potentially, at least—lead to skill and finesse in the art of making love.

Patience can also be one of the perks of a certain age. Ironically, although our biological calendars may have fewer pages left to flip, we gain a deepening awareness that there's no need to hurry, that we have all the time in the world.

Everything we have discussed thus far about the power of words, the quality of kindness, and the cultivation of a shared sense of purpose becomes amplified a hundredfold in the milieu of romance. And yet it needn't be complicated. It can be as simple as the connection created by the touch of a hand.

Through the Skin and Inward

Physical touch is an amazing bond. Thousands of nerve endings reside in a single fingertip—afferent receptors that pick up signals from the ones we touch and convey them to the brain, and efferent neurons that communicate the toucher's care and intentions outward. Millions more nerve receptors are distributed throughout the skin, which is the largest organ in the human body. Dozens of scientific studies, conducted by such prestigious medical institu-

. . . .

SMOOTH SAILING

As we get older (or, as we prefer to think of it, less obviously young), dryness of the skin and membranes becomes more of a challenge to physical intimacy. There are numerous commercial lubricants and massage oils that address this; we recommend simply keeping a little coconut oil on your night table, for a satiny and more sensual relationship. It's one of those helpful tips that can help make life pleasurable in the Second Act, and still more so in the Third.

. . . .

tions as Harvard, Duke, and the University of Miami, have demonstrated the positive effects of touch and massage on conditions ranging from colic to hyperactivity, from diabetes to migraines. Conversely, the absence of touch between a mother and child is so critical that it can retard normal growth in infants. Loving touch has been shown to stimulate pain-reducing endorphins.[32] Not that it's all about neurology, but perhaps that's one reason why a hug from Mom can make the boo-boo better, and why high blood pressure or a rapid heart rate can respond so favorably at times to a sincere hand on a shoulder.

Massage and touch have been an important component of the parenting styles in our families for decades. Our children and grandchildren have learned to heal one another with acupressure points, with a gentle hand placed on an aching head, or by firmly kneading sore muscles into suppleness. They also know to do so only with permission, as everyone's sensitivity is unique. There is no place in any relationship for coercion or control.

In different ways, the efficacy of caring touch extends also into the private relationships of intimate partners. Although this book is neither a bodywork manual nor a guide to physical intimacy, we will share here something significant we have learned.

Touch is way more than skin-deep. Beneath the surface of the body there are muscles and blood vessels, connective tissues and bones, and passageways and channels through which energy and information flow. More importantly, between all these various structures and substances there are empty spaces. We would encourage you, as you share the loving, healing, life-affirming power of touch with one another, to visualize all these internal constituents, right down to the marrow, but especially to pay attention to the empty spaces and fill them with affection, positive intention, respect, and esteem.

The Eyes of the Beholder

Speaking of visualization, a word about the eyes. Some of us are more visually oriented than others, but all of us try to forge a strong connection between what we consider beautiful and what we want. "The eye sees," the sages of antiquity say, "and the heart desires."

In modern times we have been exposed to such an overwhelming barrage of provocative images of hot models and "perfect" physiques that we sometimes forget that there are people whose bodies are beautiful, although not according to today's societally accepted stereotypes. It is not helpful to mourn the fact that you don't look anything like those magnificent specimens in the magazine ads anymore (if in fact you ever did; and you probably didn't). Because we are self-conscious and competitive, our perceived imperfections can often stand in the way of openness and relaxed intimacy.

The late Joan Rivers once quipped, "For me the best form of birth control is going to bed with the light on." Funny. We'd suggest, however, that the best way to ensure genuine intimacy might be going to bed with the light *off*.

LOOKING GOOD

Getting older doesn't mean looking grungier. Check yourself out in the mirror. Guys, is your hair combed and your shirt buttoned in the right buttonholes? Why not throw out those sweatpants with the hole in the most uncomplimentary place? Ladies, put on a little lipstick or a touch of fragrance. Keep a wardrobe well stocked with feminine nightwear, and save your baggy sports jersey for the gym. When someone is important to you, you are attentive to the impression you make. If you walk around the house looking unkempt or uncared for, you're sending a subtle message that he or she is not worthy of your honor. But keep priorities straight: remember that he cares more about the way you look at him than the way you look.

The combination of tactile connection through touch and the intoxicating power of imagination makes room for a level of pleasure and affection that cellulose, potbellies, stretch marks, and veins can sometimes impede. When you are close to someone you love in the illuminated world of possibilities that only darkness can offer, the mind will apply fond memories and kind deeds to the task of photoshopping your partner into the prince or princess charming of your heart's desire.

Keep in mind that as the years go by, it is important to accept the changes that occur in our bodies and to be aware that our intimate needs and appetites may change as well. As we mature, we often become more sensitized to a certain inherent spiritual preference for modesty in our behavior. On the other hand, some awaken to a taste for something new and different. You may think you know what your mate prefers, because that's what he or she has always responded to in the past. But don't count on it. It is helpful to be able to give and receive open, judgment-free feedback on what feels right and what does not.

Though it's incontrovertible that "nighttime is the right time" for intimate activities, there's nothing wrong with an occasional subtle allusion to your keen anticipation in the middle of the day. The mind begins to spin a web of imagination, like a computer program running in the background while you attend on screen to the tasks at hand. On a visceral level, it affords you the luxury of quietly savoring the last time you were together, and subconsciously looking forward to more. Choose a night; strategize, like young couples who can't wait for their next intimate rendezvous. Plan to be in bed by nine instead of eleven. That way you won't need to pretend you're not too tired.

Remember that the physical relationship is a gateway to emotional connection, which in turn will ripen into spiritual resonance. The innermost desire of every couple is fulfilled when two people, while evolving independently as distinct individuals, discover that they are one.

Sweating the Small Stuff

Intimacy can bring a couple to extraordinary heights of shared sensibilities and mutual openness. You may have

TIME OUT

Sometimes the best thing we can do for our relationship is to take a vacation, to reset our intention and cultivate deeper mutual appreciation. After many years or multiple decades of married life, romance can be overshadowed or overwhelmed by the rough spots.

A change of scenery or a breath of culturally fresh air can effect inner change as well. Go somewhere new, either globally or locally, for a couple of weeks if you can, or just for a night if that's what works for now. It needn't be far. A nice nearby hotel will do, as long as it's off your beaten path. Even a short staycation can reignite the magic if you approach it as an adventure. Set the mood, with candles, perhaps, or a scented bath. Open a bottle of fine wine; read to each other from poetry or inspiring prose; or perhaps watch a movie that is at once romantic and edifying, preferably with a healthy dose of redeeming intellectual or aesthetic value. Be there together and forget that anything or anyone else exists in the world. Take your time; let go of expectations.

seen some version of that cute slogan that re-frames *intimacy* as *into-me-see*—an opportunity to see deeply into your mate's heart and soul. Such peak experiences don't suddenly appear from out of the blue. They emerge as a result of everyday effort, the cumulative effect of small steps in good directions. Gestures of kindness and appreciation chip away at our default feelings of separateness and bring

CRUNCH TIME KEGELS

Exercise is a topic we'll cover in some depth in chapter 14. But one particular set of exercises bears mentioning here, as it can enhance the experience of intimacy, for him and for her, by maximizing muscle tone and the flow of blood circulation in the right areas. Known as "Kegels," these alternating contractions and relaxations of the pubococcygeal (PC) muscles of the pelvic floor should be performed for a few minutes each time, multiple times daily. It may take up to a few months to see dramatic results, but it's well worth it. For men, Kegels can prevent prostate problems and help improve erectile function. For women, they can reverse a tendency to urinary incontinence and enrich sexual pleasure immeasurably. A quick Internet search will reveal ample sources of how-to instructions for this simple and effective technique.

us closer together. It might be a word of endorsement that says, "Hey, I noticed what you did there—nice." It could be an acknowledgment of how your partner heroically suppressed a cutting remark or sarcastic retort (he or she might not see it as heroic, but you do!). Perhaps you reach out to touch his hand, for no particular reason, as he walks by on his way to the refrigerator; maybe you walk up behind her while she's cutting vegetables and surprise her with a peck on the cheek. While you're at it, offer to peel and dice the onions.

Sadly, many people are less affectionate when their stress levels are high. Precisely when a little tenderness might facilitate a welcome release of stress, we tend to stiffen and distance ourselves, exacerbating an already tense situation. Feeling uptight, hassled, overwhelmed, miffed, or preoccupied with a problem? Rather than withdrawing, try reaching out to your loved one for a simple, wordless touch or hug.

Keeping it romantic takes work, especially when you've been together for what seems like forever. But it is vital work, because the physical relationship is a key component in sustaining a vibrant level of affection and warmth.

Here too it's essential to be aware of inherent differences, which are (not necessarily, but often) a function of differences in gender. For most men, sex nourishes emotional intimacy, so the more sex they have, the more they are likely to enjoy long conversations, share feelings, use endearing language, or even snuggle. For women it is frequently the reverse—the conversation has to come first. The more women are wooed with sweet words of love, the more they feel emotionally satisfied and intellectually respected, the more likely it is that they will be amenable to sensual experience.

But it can just as easily go the other way—again, especially as we grow older and more given to role reversal. No two couples are the same in this regard, so no standardized script or magic formula holds for all. We need to keep our antennae up, become ever more aware of our spouse's internal rhythms, and do our best to ensure that both emotional intimacy and physical sex are well balanced and well timed.

Pay attention. Strive for transparency and authentic connection. Concentrate on each other. It's the secret to reclaiming yourselves as individuals, as well as partners. As we'll see in the next chapter, the benefits will accrue to ensuing generations: the happier and more devoted we are as partners, the more effective we're likely to be in our roles as matriarchs and patriarchs.

⟪ 11 ⟫

Adult Children, Children's Children, and Inner Children

Conscience is a mother-in-law whose visit never ends.

—H. L. MENCKEN

We didn't raise them to own or control them. Our intention (conscious or otherwise) in birthing and nurturing our kids was always to eventually kiss them good-bye and send them off into the world. From their perspective, they did their best to train us in the fine art of letting them go, whether by heading off to camp or to college, challenging or shattering our expectations, or simply starting families of their own. They grow, they stretch, they learn to think and fend for themselves.

Then they come home. Maybe for an hour or a day or a week, which is wonderful. Or sometimes they show up with luggage and stay for several years. In fact, the trend of millennials returning home to live with the parents they'd once left behind has become so commonplace, a special word has been coined for them: *boomerangs*. Which makes us boomers with boomerangs. Boom, boom! Sounds like a pretty explosive situation. How do we handle it? Even if they don't move in, they can be a handful. And they're no longer the little ones we once knew.

Choose Your Battles

Adult children, as much as they may admire and respect us, also look to us to respect and accept them. So we need to be sensitive to that dynamic. Don't (repeat: *don't*) tell them what to do. You can offer them information, either directly or indirectly, without making it personal or appearing judgmental. You might just leave a pertinent article lying around or discuss a given topic with your spouse or friends in front of them, rather than addressing them directly. Sometimes, in a moment of closeness and calm, and where a particularly open relationship prevails, you could ask permission to share some advice or an opinion with them. But don't offer unsolicited advice. You may well be motivated by selfless love and concern, but even well-intentioned words can easily morph into a violation of an age-old boundary.

So find your inner calm and just be. Your actions are worth ten thousand words, and your values will be communicated by osmosis. Model for them the important things: joy, kindness, tolerance, integrity, self-care, service, and respect. The natural bond between parent and child is far greater than we might imagine. Your offspring watch you closely, if sometimes casually. They notice your behavior and resonate to your tone. The choices you make, even the least significant, affect them on a deep spiritual level. Having the confidence and faith to know that you are responsible for *your* actions, not theirs, is liberating and empowering for both parent and child.

Real situations sometimes call for decisive actions, but that doesn't mean you need to be in control. Choose your battles when you must; then disarm yourself. Avoid

. . . .

A ROLE MODEL'S ROLE MODEL

During the time when I was raising my young family, I was fortunate to have as a mentor an amazing woman who came from a celebrated family of community activists (they were spiritual giants as well). I once asked her how her parents had managed to raise five children who were not only esteemed leaders in various cities around the world, but who each embodied such remarkable integrity and grace. She replied that her parents never told her or her siblings what to do— they just were who they were.

Years later, as a high school principal, I spent the majority of my time out of my office, walking the halls and dropping in on classes. Remembering my former mentor's words, I discovered that I didn't have to say much. Often just showing up was enough to influence the quality of education.

I thought of myself as an empty police car parked on the side of the road. People see the police car and slow down. That kind of quiet authority takes work to cultivate, but it's inner work. You learn to be who you be.

—Frumma

. . . .

confrontation and criticism (even if it is constructive). Remember that it is in the nature of adult children to reject your uninvited advice, in the interest of preserving their self-image and independence. Don't underestimate your influence, but examine ways in which you can convey your message simply by representing what it stands for. Often your silent presence or your understated actions will have an impact, without necessitating an uncomfortable discussion or a long-winded argument that is not likely to succeed.

Establishing Family Rituals

If you want to go beyond merely being present—if you feel your family is cohesive and trusting enough—household rituals can set the tone and facilitate effective guidance. In chapter 3 we introduced the significance of personal rituals, including the daily practice of expressing gratitude. Sometimes we can engineer ways to make that happen as a family. An ideal time might be at family dinners, when everyone is gathered together enjoying good food and an upbeat mood. In our extended family we make it a point to do so regularly, whether on Sabbaths or birthdays or when someone has just returned from a journey. We'll go around the table, taking turns, each person sharing one event or insight for which he or she is grateful. Some of our kids live far away from us, and from one another, but we still manage to get together once or twice a year. And they actually look forward to those "contrived" moments of cheerful group therapy.

The ideal time to establish such rituals is when the kids are young, but it's never too late—not even in your Third Act, when family gatherings are likely to be fewer and farther between. Think back: your family probably did follow certain kinds of rituals in its formative years, though they may have been less obvious, more unspoken. Virtually every domestic environment develops rhythmic patterns of behavior, such as how long it's acceptable to leave dirty dishes on the table, whether jackets or shoes ought to be put away in a closet, or what time of night it's too late to call. Family members internalize such expectations just by virtue of sharing the same space.

So it's not such a stretch to take it a step further and proactively introduce a new ritual or two. Some may find your suggestions hokey, but as an elder, you might find you can elicit compliance (and even score points) with ideas that never would have passed muster back when you were a highly stressed, forty-something parent of moody adolescents.

A MOMENT OF SILENCE

Here's one ritual we love. We suspect it might just be disarming enough that your family members will take to it too. What would it look like if everyone in your family knew how to step back from a tense moment, and instead of piling on one another in escalating conflict, connect with a calm inner center?

A moment of silence can be the key, and you can be the catalyst. Not by preaching to them about meditation or prayer, but by simply modeling the practice, non-invasively, by making it an I-message instead of a you-message: "I have decided that an occasional moment of silence will make me a more positive and mindful person. How great would it be if you were to support me in this initiative so I can make it stick?"

Some families can only handle this sort of thing when it's spontaneous and surprising. Others might get into it as a more regularly scheduled exercise, however brief, of reflection or emotional release. One of Simcha's daughters reminds her child to take a deep breath when he begins to work himself up over whatever triviality happens to be hijacking his nervous system. It has become a staple feature of family behavior management, and it works. As the kids grow older, such moments will acquire more meaning. Self-control becomes a no-brainer when it emerges out of an internalized awareness that we are always free to choose how we will respond to situations.

It Takes a Tribe

One of the unfortunate side effects of modern life is that older and younger generations tend to live separate lives. Once upon a time, elders and young'uns lived in close proximity, if not under the same roof. It worked to everyone's advantage. The kids were doted on by loving grandparents and gained some appreciation for the wisdom that accrues from life experience. And the older generation stayed young at heart, and kept their knees in shape

. . . .

PRETTY FLY FOR A GRANDMA

A five-year-old was asked where his grandma lives. "Oh that's easy," he said. "She lives at the airport, and when we want her, we just go get her. Then, when we've talked enough, we bring her back to the airport."

. . . .

by gleefully crawling around on the floor after toddlers. We're not advocating a return to such apparently idyllic times—we do manage to see the upside when the grandkids go home by bedtime—but there's much to be learned from this "tribal" approach. Even if it's just for a Sunday barbecue or a weekend sleepover, spending quality multigenerational time together on a regular basis enriches our lives immeasurably.

It does take some effort (not to mention some sagacity) to reap the benefits. To elicit a spirit of cooperation and harmony is far from automatic, especially in the presence of the inevitable tensions that can arise in any family's dynamic. As the senior members of the team, we are uniquely positioned to keep the communication open and flowing. The foundation of that expertise lies first in knowing, with all the certainty we can summon, that everyone wants to be a useful, generous, valued contributor to the common cause, whether or not they are willing to admit it at first.

Service is one of the languages of love. We are here not just to give back but to give unconditionally. As true as that may be in the universe at large, it's even more real and tangible in our microcosmic homes. Where better to practice being a happy giver than in our own kitchens and living rooms?

Ironically, however, sometimes we don't succeed in conveying a spirit of loving collaboration because we fail to establish boundaries and put limits on our own big hearts. That's when a loving parent crosses a line and begins to play the role of the martyr: always giving, always serving, supremely responsible . . . and secretly resentful.

Our adult children know us well enough to sense the negativity that we imagine we have successfully masked. They would be much more comfortable with an honest, "I don't want to handle all this myself. What would you like to do to help?"

....

THE GOOD LIFE?

If you think fame and fortune are the keys to human happiness, think again.

Dr. Robert Waldinger is a professor of clinical psychiatry and the director of the Harvard Study of Adult Development. He and his team have tracked data over a span of seventy-five years to evaluate the most significant factors that lead to health and well-being as we age. It's the longest study of its kind ever done, and the results are definitive and unequivocal.

"Good relationships," Dr. Waldinger attests, "keep us happier and healthier. Period."

....

Also solicit their opinions and advice. They want to know that you value their intelligence, ideas, and experience. Often their new and youthful outlook will help you to grow and improve the quality of your life.

We do this with our grandchildren. It closes the generation gap and opens up fresh areas of opportunity. Like the time we were away in the mountains on a writing retreat, discovered we had no Internet service, and desperately needed to back up our writing to the cloud. We are fairly tech-savvy for a couple of geezers, but it was only by the good graces of a grandchild that we figured out how to use a cell phone as a hot spot and gain access to the Internet. Our children love being our teachers, and we love when they clue us in to the latest, hippest selection of microbrew beers, a great practical suggestion from a website we hadn't seen, or some amazing new music. (Yes, the oldies were great. But beware of sounding like your parents when they'd say to you, wincing in pain, "You call that music?")

Tips for Dealing with Adult Children

It is essential to keep growing, and wonderful to keep growing together. Listening to your children's ideas also paves the way for offering some sage counsel of our own, in those situations where we feel we must. *Seven Habits* author Stephen Covey writes about the importance of investing in what he calls an "emotional bank account." You make deposits by spending quality time with them, giving positive strokes or hands-on help, or offering useful gifts that demonstrate how you get who they are. Being open-minded and listening attentively to what your kids have to say will also add value. All these deposits build your bank balance, so that when you need to make a withdrawal, such as in discussing a sensitive issue or setting a personal boundary they may not like, you have surplus funds to cover it.[33]

Here are some additional emotional investment tips for those always delicate, ever-so-rewarding relationships with adult children:

- When there's a disagreement, be willing to let go. The more objective and the less invested you are in being right, the more likely you'll be heard. That doesn't mean roll over and give up. Just don't take it personally if they don't accept your perspective. They're not rejecting *you*.

- If particular behaviors are bothering you, try to understand why. Often it's because they remind you of yourself. Perhaps it is more in the interest of peace, progress, and your own self-refinement for you to forgo the judgment.

- Avoid temperamental language like "you always" do this or "you never" do that. Such phrases are generally an exaggeration and a source of stress. They tend to eclipse the times when it wasn't so and deter the positive changes you seek.

- Be curious. Ask questions. Whether as a parent, a coach, a healer or an educator, giving top-down advice is rarely effective. By asking them what they think and want rather than telling them what they *ought* to want, you endow your adult children with independence. They will more readily invest in the solutions they come up with, because they own them.

∾ Timing is key. Don't try to appease your adult child when she's in a rage or press her to accept consolation when her heart has just broken. Take your time. Call upon your inner calm and try to feel what they're feeling. Refrain from confrontation in the heat of a moment; wait for an opening before opening your mouth. Sometimes it's smart to rehearse what you are going to say. You might role-play a difficult conversation first with a friend. Be mindful of your tone of voice. Root out words that might be heard as judgments.

∾ Accentuate the positive, but try to stay away from broad, sweeping compliments or overly sweet optimism. Instead, be specific. Describe some particular aspect of what you see happening that gives you a reason to be happy or proud. Acknowledge the good and express it verbally. But don't oversell it. Why invite resistance?

∾ If your married child is complaining about his or her spouse, never agree with the criticism, even if you're so inclined. The couple will most likely make up and forget about it, but your child will continue to remember what you said.

In-laws or Outlaws?

The challenge of peaceful coexistence with our own children often pales in comparison with the complications of relationships between in-laws. Naturally it's far more difficult to establish an adult-child relationship with someone else's adult child. You've spent years making hefty deposits in your own children's emotional bank accounts; with these new kids on the block, you're starting with a more or less blank slate. It's a complex dance, fraught with pitfalls.

Not to minimize the awkwardness that can exist between a father and his son-in-law, but it's the mother-in-law/daughter-in-law relationship (MIL/DIL for short) that is usually the most troublesome. Can two women love the same man and peacefully coexist?

Mother-in-law jokes are a mainstay of comedy. Most of them play on the stereotype that characterizes the average mother-in-law as overbearing, obnoxious, and unattractive to boot. Most significantly, the old battle-ax considers her daughter-in-law to be absolutely unworthy of her son. Needless to say, such feelings are readily reciprocated. The Internet abounds with "I hate my mother-in-law" websites.

Unfortunately—one might even say tragically—our contemporary society has by and large ceased to understand the value of extended family. This is particularly true of the MIL/DIL relationship. "Love your neighbor as yourself," we tell ourselves. "Judge everyone favorably; give them the benefit of the doubt." Yet when it comes to sticky, hypersensitive MIL/DIL moments, there can be more doubt than benefit. Daughters-in-law are rarely comfortable enough to engage in open communication with their mothers-in-law, let alone accept their well-considered advice. Conversely, mothers-in-law, convinced it's for the good of the family,

SOLOMON'S CHOICE

Two mothers appear before King Solomon, the wisest of all men. Each one claims that a certain young man has pledged his troth to her daughter. King Solomon decides: cut the man in half, and they'll each have a piece of him.

"Oh, no!" cries the first woman, "Please, let him live!"

"No problem," says the second, "Cut him in half!"

"Aha!" exclaims the king. "The second one is the true mother-in-law!"

will eagerly intervene, utterly blind to the resistance and resentment their unwelcome criticism engenders. Discomfort turns to judgment, which before long gives way to paranoia, and the MIL/DIL syndrome is in full flower.

Totally overlooked is the fact that the MIL/DIL relationship is potentially the most fertile partnership a family could cultivate. These two lucky ladies would have worlds to offer each other, if only they could overcome their hang-ups and negativity to work and play well together. A mother-in-law ought to honor and appreciate the woman who will care for her son's spiritual, physical, and emotional needs for the rest of his life. She needs to train herself to look upon her daughter-in-law with a "good eye," seeing the good in her and ditching the judgment.

By the same token, a daughter-in-law should try to value and welcome her mother-in-law's wisdom, concern, and in-the-trenches experience with the man they both love. In the interest of true mutual growth, we can work on surrendering our defensiveness. When a girl leaves her childhood home to join her husband's "tribe," who can best enhance the bride's understanding of his well-worn ways?

In education, it's called professionalism: third-grade teachers end a school year by meeting with the fourth-grade teachers, filling them in on the strengths and weaknesses of their future students. In business transactions, it's called common sense: an educated consumer buying a used car solicits the advice of the previous owner, to learn the vehicle's quirks and what the new owner should do to maintain it. Perhaps the groom has a few idiosyncrasies that his wife hasn't yet figured out; maybe her mother-in-law can fill in the missing links. By the way, it's entirely possible that a new wife will have insights to offer that his mother may have missed.

Yet how often do a MIL and DIL create opportunities to optimize the transition, to bond in a way that will establish peace in the home and transmit sound values from one generation to the next? Are we ready for the internal work it takes to transform uneasiness into continuity, loyalty, and love? Why not take walks in the park together, or do lunch, just the two of us, and listen, and learn?

As the more mature member of this twosome, it behooves the mother-in-law to take the first steps toward such a loving and productive relationship. MILs and DILs have so much in common. You both want only the best for

THE Q-TIP

We need tools to cultivate the MIL/DIL relationship. Here's one we often offer to clients and friends: the Q-TIP, as in "Quit Taking It Personally." If the DIL is too busy to invite you into her life, let go of your umbrage. Maybe you can replace your irritation at having been slighted with a positive resolve to help her have more free time. Offer to run one of her carpools, perhaps, or slip her a few twenties, if you have the means, for extra cleaning help. And in those inevitable moments when helpful suggestions or offers of time, service, an extra set of hands, or even money are met with resistance, let it pass.

your guy, and for the future of the family—happiness, good health, positive communication, and financial and physical well-being. Not to mention a sense of belonging, purpose, integrity, and continuity.

From a broader perspective than that of our own personal agendas, our daughters-in-law and sons-in-law are precisely as they "should" be (as are, by the way, our spouses, children, and grandchildren). In releasing our tenacious grip on our own personal territory—our script, our control, our point of view—we expand our consciousness and grow more whole. We become adept at loving all family members for who they are. They, and we, are freed to become all we are capable of being. And this sets the tone for generations to come.

If We Knew How Wonderful Grandchildren Were Going to Be, We'd Have Had Them First

We love grandchildren with the same love we feel for our children, but without the burdens of responsibility, without the pressures, the urgency, and the guilt. There is something mature and disentangled in the way we care for them. Their parents, our kids, outgrew their diapers and braces, their acne and awkwardness, their rowdiness and rebellion. So we have the experience and the insight to trust that the grandkids will too. We understand that we can give them tools, information, and opportunities, but we can't make their decisions for them or put their resources to work. As grandparents we have the luxury of being less preoccupied with their day-to-day physical health and safety than their parents need to be, and more concerned with their long-term sense of destiny and the well-being of their souls.

There is a wealth of print and online information on grandparenting. These articles and books focus almost exclusively on how to keep in touch and make grandparenting fun, from clever intergenerational arts and crafts projects to entertaining daytrips and vacations. But grandparenting is much more than that. We have a legacy to share with them. At a certain point in their development, they begin to realize that they look to us to be wise as well as fun.

Even before that happy moment arrives, we can start sowing seeds. We can play ball with them, go Rollerblading if our knees can handle that, or bond with them over spectator sports if not. Even better, we can also use those opportunities to speak about good sportsmanship, to imbue competitive games with a measure of social intelligence. We can show them that we are with-it enough to appreciate the latest dance steps or hip-hop lyrics, yet make that a vehicle for sharing with them the more sophisticated pleasures of the classics. We can tell them about their roots, show them pictures of their parents when they were young, laugh with them over the funny stuff mom or dad used to do. We can plant a garden, or an idea.

Thanks to the marvels of technology, we can be a different brand of grandparent than ever existed before. We can send them email or texts, chat with them on Face-Time, and friend them on Facebook. But the dignity of the wise patriarch or matriarch should not be taken lightly. A grandparent's guidance has an extra quality that supplements and enhances parental influence. While mom and dad are necessarily focused on the pragmatics of dinner-times and dental floss, we have a unique edge in sensitizing our grandchildren to the finer things in life.

The quality we bring to the table is more spiritual, less mired in the practical aspects of getting through the tough times. Our guidance flows from a place of life experience, of survival-against-the-odds. The judgment-free nature of the grandparent-grandchild bond makes us uniquely suited to the awesome project of marinating our grandkids in unconditional love.

When you speak with a grandchild, you can indulge in the sort of language of the spirit that might induce eye rolling on the part of their parents. Using words like *loving*,

PRECIOUS MOMENTS IN NATURE

Natural beauty opens windows on a transcendent realm that is far beyond words, offering awe-filled experiences we can share with our grandchildren. Not long ago we experienced a magnificent mountain sunset up at the end of a winding trail. There were no people or architectural artifacts there to mar the lush landscape, the impressionistic array of wildflowers, the blazing sky darkening into cottony shades of gold and blue and black. Humanity seemed so small, and creation so majestic. We didn't speak. Neither did the kids.

Some children will relish such moments; most are more drawn to bright lights, little pixels, and hasty games. With them, the photos on our phones might have to suffice until they're ready for more tranquil pleasures. But with intention and planning, we can enjoy amazing moments in nature with each grandchild, individually. It is something we owe them.

adoring, enduring, considerate, kindhearted, or *compassionate,* you can transport the little ones from a world of carpools, homework, and orthodontists to a less frenetic reality. Your deliberate use of more lyrical language can turn their thoughts from superheroes, trading cards, and terrorists to sages, angels, and holy men. (OK, probably not every grandchild. Some will respond; some won't. But those who don't will feel your sincerity anyway.)

Proudly but humbly take your place as their spiritual role model. Let them know that our actions as individuals have an impact on the universe and that the world is built on lovingkindness. Inspire them with the idea that there is an Eye that sees and an Ear that hears, and they are accountable for their deeds. Demonstrate your integrity by making an additional effort to be kind, pleasant, upbeat, and giving when you are around them. Avoid speaking negatively about people. Instead express gratitude; share a story about something nice that happened to you or someone you know.

Your grandchildren will notice your attention to ethical behavior. They'll remember if you paid the correct admission price at the theme park or the aquarium, observed the speed limit, cleaned up your messes, recycled in public places, or showed concern for the welfare of animals. Watching you perform acts of kindness and charity, they will be touched. Seeing your love of justice, they will grow.

There is a longstanding tradition (and we've seen this often among our circle of friends) that grandparents are more likely than parents to pass on religious beliefs and spiritual practices to their grandchildren. Mom and Dad are often preoccupied with the worldly pursuits of livelihood and practical parenthood. They may also have been influenced by contemporary trends of diminishing involvement in organized religion, or more inclined toward a self-defined sense of spirituality than institutional forms of worship. Even if they are churchgoers or members of a mosque or synagogue, their roles vis-à-vis the kids may well be more about enforcement than inspiration.

SIMCHA GETS BEGETTING

As a child I barely knew my grandparents, and I grew up in a broken home. As a young adult, I was fortunate to know a few intact extended families, and it was something of a revelation to me to see multiple generations getting along with respect, sometimes even with reverence. None of that struck me as personally relevant, however, until I got a wake-up call from what was, for me, an unlikely source.

Up to that point whatever spiritual stirrings I had experienced were private, meditative, and untethered to any particular tradition. More or less out of nowhere, I began to dip into the scriptures of various cultures. Though it was by no means my first stop, at a certain juncture I found myself exploring those five books from Sinai that the world refers to as the Torah. I read in Genesis about the ten generations from Adam to Noah. And all of them were begetting and begetting and begetting, until the planet was teeming with life. Then things didn't turn out so well; but all of a sudden here came ten more generations, from Noah to Abraham—and again with the begetting. There was something about that I liked, and I wanted in.

The rest, as they say, is history, but here's my point: we are defined not so much by our individual lives (though each of those is priceless too) but by our generations, by the quality of life we receive from forebears and the evolving legacies we leave. Continuity is king.

Enter Grandma and Grandpa. We can speak with them about matters of the spirit in the caring, patient way of a patriarch or matriarch. We can ask them their opinions as well and entertain their questions. You can even luxuriate in discussing the subtleties of faith and the sublime power of love, if that's your bag. At the very least we can hang out with them in the kitchen preparing something special for a holiday meal, or singing traditional songs, or reading together from a book of prayers or stories or scriptures. Whatever floats your mutual boat.

Why do grandparents and grandchildren get along so well? We venture to suggest that it's because we have similar relationships with the eternal cycle of life, or what philosophers like to call the "arrow of time." Kids are closer to the beginning of their sojourn in this world; elders are becoming ever more aware of their own mortality. Both, therefore, are gifted with opportunities to embrace the present moment more intensely and more expansively than those who are constantly *pressed* for time, in the heat of the everyday battles they face. It's a high-quality relationship with what's happening *now*, and *now*, and *now*. Or as we referred to it in an earlier chapter in another context, *affluence of time*. Young children and their aging grandparents are both fabulously wealthy, in ways that the intervening generations may have (temporarily) forgotten about. The earliest melodies of the symphony of life are embedded in its last glorious choruses. How great is it when the vigor of youth and the ripened fruits of maturity come together to compose that masterwork?

Then there are times when even a well-honed sense of presence in the moment can be challenged by unforeseen, perhaps tragic events. We may be pressed into a service for which we feel unprepared, unsheltered from the storm of circumstance. When a loved one suddenly needs us, how shall we manage to keep an even keel, and fortify ourselves to keep on giving informed and effective care?

Caregivers Anonymous

Caregiving has no second agendas or hidden motives.
The care is given from love for the joy of giving
without expectations, no strings attached.
—GARY ZUKAV, AUTHOR OF *THE SEAT OF THE SOUL*

We strode confidently into adulthood, ready to face tough times, willing and able to confront the worst of times. Yet how many of us envisioned the actual eruption of catastrophe into our own lives?

Some of us took wedding vows and pledged ourselves to an everlasting bond—*for better or for worse, through sickness and in health, until the inevitable expiration of this mortal coil do us part*. And then life happens. A partner's health begins to fail. He can't perform the simple tasks you took for granted a year ago. She goes for treatments, returns home weak, increasingly dependent, or even incapacitated. Suddenly you are a caretaker, a nurse. If you can't bring yourself to embrace the role and rise to the challenge, you may feel more like a prisoner.

Some of us are accidental angels, pressed into service by a mishap that befalls a friend, an elderly parent, a sibling—and by the unforeseen awakening of our need to be needed. Or a loved one descends into what seems to be the downward spiral of degenerative disease, and our only choice is not a choice at all, but an ironclad commitment to care and be there for him or her.

At times like these, our carefree theme of *getting better all the time* begins to sound glib and unrealistic. Becoming a cheerful and enlightened caregiver is never easy, even for the most optimistic among us. Can we reframe these dark stories into a perspective that sees them as opportunities, not as burdens, and lessens the pain of tragedy? We might tell ourselves that it's our karma, that the big wheel of consequences has spun this way to remind us how what goes around comes around. We might see such events as testimony to the idealistic notion that "we live to serve," or as a test of the gratitude to which we've been paying lip service all our lives.

As in so many aspects of life, when faced with such a serious challenge, your attitude is the key to your triumph. You can embrace and accept the principle that everything happens for a reason, that a Higher Power has prescribed this for both you and the one who needs you as a means to achieve self-refinement. Or you can subscribe to the idea that everything is random, that meaning and justice are illusory. In real life many of us find ourselves influenced by both perspectives at once, or we might oscillate between them. It's not necessarily either/or. The net effect is, you have a choice: you can welcome the struggle, or you can be resentful and resistant.

However we understand (or fail to understand) the situation, it is really happening. It can be sad, or worse, and sometimes it can be really hard to handle. Here are a few tools and insights that we hope will make the experience a little richer and give you a bit more capability to cope.

In Whom Do We Trust?

Caring for those who are experiencing a diminished ability to care for themselves brings with it many challenges. Among the biggest pitfalls is one we may not think of right off the bat. It's our tendency to *over*care, to take too much responsibility.

Sometimes in our sincere and loving efforts to be protective and comforting, we run the risk of robbing our loved one of personal power. He or she needs a strong sense of self to face adversity, carry on, and make a comeback. When we feel overly protective, we can become controlling and doting, hovering like a loving helicopter, and in our well-meaning watchfulness, we may give too much.

The ironic result of this sort of excessive generosity is that we can go from being care*givers* to care*takers*. We think we are giving, but instead we are taking away our loved ones' autonomy, depriving them of the chance to strengthen themselves with self-sufficiency.

This syndrome has become commonplace in modern medicine's paternalistic culture, with its emphasis on high-tech, specialized expertise. Patients are encouraged (perhaps not intentionally, but nonetheless) to abdicate responsibility for their own health. More and more, we go running to the doctor for every ailment, even those minor afflictions that might best be treated with common sense.

> *Nothing can bring you peace but yourself. Nothing can bring you peace but the triumph of principles. Trust thyself: every heart vibrates to that iron string.*
> —RALPH WALDO EMERSON, "SELF RELIANCE"

There's been much debate about these issues among the medical profession. There is, in fact, a welcome trend toward greater emphasis on preventive medicine, better access to medical information, and encouraging people to take personal responsibility for their own wellness. But the "system" (including the insurance and pharmaceutical industries, and the market realities physicians must deal with) still tends to keep patient populations in a state of dependency.

Nonetheless, in the *non*professional realm of caregiving among loving relatives and friends, if we pay attention, we can strike a healthy balance between offering an appropriate helping hand and stepping back to allow people to help themselves.

Have an honest discussion with your loved one about the extent to which he or she feels capable of taking responsibility. Revisit that conversation as you confront together the daily decisions, large and small. As caregivers, we need to make it clear that we are there for them, yet we respect them too much to do everything for them. Be decisive when necessary, but be ready to hand them the reins. They will trust us all the more if we offer them opportunities to become more self-reliant and learn to trust themselves. Ultimately, this mutual cultivation of trust trains us all in the fine art of trusting in a higher, transcendent source of healing.

Not that we wish adversity on anyone (may we all enjoy perfect health all our days!), but illness, when it happens, can enhance our powers of introspection and trigger tremendous personal growth. Like an olive in an olive press, when we are squeezed by life's difficult circumstances, precious essence emerges.

Educating Ourselves as Caregivers

The better informed you are about your loved one's condition, the more effective care you can give. Doing the research also gives you a small sense of participation, if not control, in decisions; it can open your eyes to a wide range of options for both traditional and complementary treatment strategies. Your investigations may well unveil a realistic, customized alternative to the conventional medical approach. Numerous creative, tried-and-true ways are available to alleviate the discomforts that accompany illness and boost core vitality. Among them are such millennia-old solutions as acupuncture, herbal remedies, massage, and nutritional therapies. In many cases these and other modalities can provide viable solutions that Pfizer and Merck cannot.

Yet caution is called for, and there is no substitute for the wise guidance and clinical experience of a seasoned medical professional. Doctor Google can be a valuable consultant or a dangerous charlatan. When it comes to health and wellness, we tend to be staunch advocates of self-reliance and personal responsibility, but this must always be balanced by a measure of deference to a trusted physician who has spent a lifetime pursuing the knowledge we seek. We owe it to those we care for to help them find the best possible medical personnel.

We also may need to advocate for a loved one who suffers from diminished capacity in the corridors of a confounding, convoluted health care system. It has become increasingly common for insurers to deny coverage or place arbitrary limits on the treatments doctors are authorized to provide. For such questions, as well as regarding the legal, ethical, and religious ramifications of living wills and advance healthcare directives, Internet resources can help.[34] Where possible, however, it may prove wisest to turn first to the more personal guidance of community spiritual leaders and local service organizations.

When seeking the best physicians, how do we decide? A mentor of ours who is frequently consulted in cases of medical urgency offers an interesting rule of thumb. All other things being equal, he suggests, one should choose a "healer who is also a friend." By this he means to say that a proven track record of medical success is important, but not necessarily the whole story. You should also look for someone you know to be concerned and compassionate, who knows you and/or the patient—if not very well, then at least well enough to be able to discern the unique background, circumstances, or perspective on life that distinguishes you from the crowd. Each of us, after all, is unique. As is every physician. It is essential that there be resonance and empathy between the healer and the healed.

While we must carefully verify any medical information we discover on the Internet, some amazing resources are available online that can facilitate our quest to imbue caregiving with optimum quality. Among these are networking sites, such as www.lotsahelpinghands.com and www.takethemameal.com; and information aggregators like www.carepages.com. (Online communities are rapidly evolving, so these links may or may not be current as you are reading this, but that's what search engines are for.)

So take advantage of the emerging technologies to find emotional support or practical assistance, and broaden the scope of your caregiving. Being part of a larger network will help both of you. It can help prevent caregiver burnout, and provide you, your loved one, and your extended support group with clearer communications, greater optimism, and an enhanced ability to get things done.

Self-Care Is Also Caregiving

"This slice of bread on my plate," an old saying goes, "is yours just as much as it is mine." One of the highest expressions of human kindness—perhaps *the* highest—is the sort of selfless generosity that moves us to give, even when it hurts. Yet for kindness to be consistent and sustainable, balance is required. Man doth not live by altruism alone.

In caring for others, there are times when internal tranquility can take precedence over external productivity. Sometimes your own happiness is a prerequisite to the happiness of your loved one. Self-care, therefore, is one of the most essential ingredients in the formula for compassionate care. The word itself, *compassion*, offers us a hint in its original meaning: *com* = *with*, and *passion* = *feeling*. It means that when we *feel with* someone, we care for them *with feeling*. If you feel good, there's a good chance those around you will too.

So instead of sacrificing yourself nonstop in the service of the needs of another, be sure to take some quality time for yourself. It's not a luxury. A trip to the beach or the gym, the attention you give to eating healthy and nourishing foods, or those few moments you "steal" for meditation, uplifting cultural events, or just plain laid-back relaxation, are far from selfish. They are acts of kindness, because they will help you infuse the time you spend as a caregiver with true compassion.

This crucial lesson is embedded in the safety instructions the airlines offer as we buckle our seat belts to take off on a flight. "In the unlikely event of an emergency," we are assured, "an oxygen mask will drop down before you. Be sure to put on and adjust your own mask before attempting to assist others."

To be an effective first responder, you need to first be response-able. It's important to recognize and define your limits—to know the extent of your capabilities and avoid pushing yourself too hard, too fast. Set reasonable, incremental goals for yourself. When you achieve them, step back and breathe a bit to evaluate your next set of goals rather than driving yourself compulsively beyond your boundaries. Sometimes we keep dancing as fast as we can, only to eventually fall on our faces.

By the same token, caregivers need to learn that they can accept support from other caregivers—family, good friends, or members of our various communities. Allow yourself to delegate responsibilities to those who are willing and able to pitch in with you. Often people would like to help, but don't quite know what to do or how to make the offer. You may even be unwittingly discouraging them from offering assistance by projecting a ruggedly independent attitude that's not consistent with the way you actually feel.

Sit down with a pen and pad or a laptop; make a list of the tasks at hand and divide them up: shopping, making a meal, driving to the doctor, or simply spending time with your loved one while you grab some needed downtime. And delegate.

Here are a few more strategies for fulfilling the commandment "Thou shall not be a martyr":

- ∾ Introduce stress reduction techniques into your daily routine, such as breathing exercises or mini-meditations (for a few examples, see chapter 5).

- Find someone you can trust as a confidant for times when you need a release valve or some friendly advice—perhaps another caregiver in a similar situation, who knows the ropes and can share advice on the struggle. It's important to be able to articulate feelings, fears, or frustrations.

- Sometimes a more professional sounding board is called for, whether a therapist, social worker, life coach, or clergy member. They are trained to help you address a wide range of physical and emotional issues.

- Utilize respite care services—an amazing asset when you need a temporary break. The relief such agencies offer can range from a few hours of in-home care to brief "vacations" in a nursing home or assisted-living facility. Yes, it can be challenging to entrust your loved one to someone else's care, but sometimes you need to let go of control. It helps to do our homework first: get a few letters of reference or visit the facility and watch how they interact with their clients, and then listen to your intuition.

- Some communities boast volunteer services that include trained home health caregivers. In some towns, students need community service hours, and a local high school guidance counselor can connect you with eager young people to lend a hand, or relieve you while you run to the store.

- Join a local support group, which you can usually find through an online search. Share your feelings and experiences with other caregivers who are in a similar situation. It can help you manage stress, locate useful resources, and stay connected.

∽ Maintain a sense of humor. It's easy to get weighed down with the seriousness of it all. Interject a light moment whenever you can; do whatever seems appropriate to keep yourself and your loved one in a good mood. Never underestimate the healing power of an old Marx Brothers movie.

Traction: An Antidote for Angst

Whenever one is burdened with heavy responsibility, it's normal to experience negative feelings. Sometimes it's that voice inside that cries, "Why *me*?" You might feel overwhelmed or view yourself as a victim. You might harbor anger toward your loved one (inevitably accompanied by guilt for having the feeling) or even rage against God for placing you in this situation. It doesn't mean you're a bad person or a bad caregiver. It may mean that you're missing an opportunity to grow. And growth begins with accepting where you are and who you are, rather than succumbing to the coulda-shoulda-woulda syndrome of wishing in vain that you'd been dealt a better hand.

The art of acceptance entails the ability to realize that in the greater scheme of things, the situation you "find yourself in" is not an accident. Where you are is exactly where you are meant to be. With a little introspection and a lot of letting go you can turn adversity into a victory of

ON A FLIGHT FROM PHOENIX

Some decades ago, a buddy and I took a hiking and camping trip together to the Grand Canyon. At the time he was in the early years of his career as a family physician. I was in the somewhat shaky throes of my second or third change of profession. It was a seminal spiritual experience in both our lives, and served to deepen our friendship.

On the flight back east from Phoenix, we shared and commiserated over our respective worries and concerns. He told me about how difficult it was to be a family practitioner in a large, close-knit community, where hundreds of families felt entitled to come running to him at all hours of the day and night with their crises, aches, and pains. He resented the intrusions on his privacy, yet chastised himself for what he felt was a deficit in the generosity of spirit that had inspired his career choice in the first place. He was not fully at peace with his profession, ambivalent about the choices he'd made.

We spoke for hours, baring our souls, exploring the dual motivations of people in the helping professions: the desire to serve those in need and the seemingly self-serving desire to be needed. By the end of that flight, a certain quality of self-acceptance had set in. He had gained traction.

No doubt other life experiences turned further pages in his life. But that conversation was pivotal. A long, happy, successful career ensued, helping countless families and saving many lives.

—Simcha

your stronger, better nature over your habitual patterns of passivity, weakness, or victimhood.

We call this emotional anchoring *traction*. When the wheels of a vehicle fail to grip the road, they spin ineffectually and go nowhere. If the left foot isn't firmly planted on the ground, the right leg cannot stride forward. In accepting the perfectness of the imperfection that is, we gain the power to work on our surroundings and ourselves. With traction, we gain command of our vision. With a fine blend of equanimity and perseverance, we can then proceed to transform the realities we face.

We're not suggesting that gaining traction is easy or automatic, that just by snapping our fingers and saying, "Got it!" we actually get it. Getting it takes some internal exertion.

GRATITUDE REDUX

We've spoken earlier in this book about the power of gratitude. We've recommended making lists of things we appreciate or keeping a daily gratefulness notebook (see chapter 3). Here we want to emphasize that training ourselves to see what's good about our current situation and striving to cultivate warm feelings of appreciation are keys to gaining traction. Even when it's hard to breathe, let alone feel good, we can find *something* positive and feel it. From there it becomes a matter of making this process a habit, of growing these good feelings organically inside, until gratitude grows and climbs over the obstacles in our lives.

One last anecdote will help solidify our points on gratitude. A male friend was hospitalized with a terminal illness. He was determined to maintain a positive attitude and a pleasant countenance toward his loved ones, though that was not his normal nature. He decided that the best way to achieve this was through a gratitude journal. So he asked his wife to bring him a pen and a notebook. The next morning, at a bit of a loss as to what to include in the journal, he decided he would express his appreciation for the next individual who entered his room.

Before long, an orderly entered the room with a cup of midmorning coffee. It was the usual mediocre hospital fare, but he wrote pages on the kindness and professionalism of the hospital staff, the hard labor of the coffee growers and processors, the amazing selection of coffees available in local specialty shops, the steps necessary to plant and refine the sugar and feed and milk the cow, the advent of pasteurization, and even the practical utility of the Styrofoam cup in which the coffee was served. When he was finished, he had composed twenty pages of gratitude for a lousy cup of coffee as he lay dying in a hospital bed.

His caregivers were astounded. Having learned a priceless lesson from him, as time passed they were able to share that lesson and enrich the lives of others; and they in turn continued to find their own lives enriched by those for whom they cared.

But what happens when someone to care for is missing in our lives, and we find ourselves not only alone, but lonely?

~ 13 ~

Single at Sixtysomething

Sometimes I wish I could jump into the dryer and
come out wrinkle-free and a few sizes smaller.
—SPOTTED ON A PARK BENCH IN OXNARD, CALIFORNIA

Call us crazy, but one of our favorite venues for gaining flashes of insight into other people is the local supermarket. It's one of the few places where people from totally disparate walks of life share the same public space and move slowly enough to be seen. As a couple of ex-foodies (OK, maybe the "ex" part is not entirely honest), we take particular delight in watching perfect strangers interact with their meal plans.

Every once in a while we do the grocery shopping together rather than running individual errands. Somehow doubling the work force frees us up to notice more about our fellow shoppers. We see the harried mom with three little ones in tow, exercising the wisdom of Solomon in every aisle while the kids whine, cajole, and blackmail her for treats she'd rather they didn't have; the camp counselor filling up his cart with two-liter soda bottles and jumbo bags of chips; the dutiful husband with his nose in his shopping list; the prudent homemaker studying lists of ingredients; the couch potatoes in tank tops debating over which six-packs to buy. You can learn a lot under those too-bright fluorescent lights, with soft classic rock barely audible in the background.

The other day, our cart overflowing with provisions for an impending weekend with extended, blended family swooping into town, we happened to peek into the hand-held shopping basket of a sweet older lady in the checkout line next to ours. Her purchase consisted of two bananas, one tomato, a frozen entrée, and some cat food. She had a tranquil, patient look about her. Her eyes, slightly down-cast, did not budge, neither to the right or the left.

We're not so presumptuous as to assume we got this exactly right, but at that moment it appeared to us that we had caught a glimpse into the quintessential loneliness of age.

Loneliness comes in many forms. Some people can feel isolated and alone in a room full of people. Others experience loneliness when separated from friends or family, even if only temporarily. When the stories of our lives have advanced into their Third Acts, many of us find ourselves suddenly unattached or undernourished by human contact. Aloneness may be the result of a breakup, or a debilitating illness, or the death of a spouse. Sometimes a lifelong history of uneasy relationship can metastasize over time into irreconcilable differences, and what was once a partnership comes undone.

Children grow up and leave home; the house is tidier, but quieter. Children move to other coasts or continents, or their spouses are uncomfortable with us, and visits are fewer and farther between. Friends pass away, mates leave the world; PTA meetings and carpools and workplace social interactions have become a thing of the past.

Time heals many wounds, they say, and all sorts of pain can pass. But some loneliness isn't temporary and isn't likely to change with time. Even with the advent of a new job or a new grandbaby, the loneliness of age won't disappear. Because it's not about circumstances. At its core, it's not even contingent upon whether or not we are in the presence of loved ones or socially connected.

Redefining Loneliness

The inner loneliness of the soul is not inherently sad. In its essence, it can be infused with delight: it's that wonderful singularity that defines the unique individuality of every human being. But with advancing age, one can fall into anxiety, brought on by the inexorable advance toward the end of our sojourn here—that culminating gateway through which each one of us will pass alone. This fear can only be healed by a conscious, internal shift in perspective. We must apprehend the aloneness and transform it before it transforms us.

We can begin by renaming it. We can redefine *loneliness* as glorious *solitude*. Instead of a curse, it becomes a gift, an opportunity to spend our hours and days in walking meditation, as though we are on permanent vacation on an imaginary beach or in metaphorical mountains. This newfound sense of sweet solitude affords us the quietude to think straight, to internalize the lessons we have accumulated over the years. When we reframe it well, it can become a deep inhalation of fresh air. Having renamed it, we can embark upon the redemptive process of transforming feelings of loneliness into a fully charged sense of independence.

On the other hand, no one is an island; even an adamant introvert craves connection at times. Then there are those among us who can't live comfortably without a healthy measure of social interaction. We'll revisit the power of solitude before this chapter's done, but for now let's have a look at how to deal with those inevitable moments when its just not OK to be alone. Sometimes we need to put ourselves out there and meet people.

The Extrovert's Dilemma

When a person has spent the better part of a lifetime cultivating meaningful long-term relationships, artificial meet-and-greet events can be painful. Real friendships unfold over time, based on shared experiences, building trust, and the weeding out of fair-weather friends. Common interests may indicate the possibility of genuine affinity, but there's nothing automatic about the process of discovering resonance and acquiring a friend.

Nonetheless, we have to start somewhere. Even a contrived way of coming out of a cocoon can be better than none. If you like the outdoors, you might join a hiking club or find a local cycling or golfing group. Some will prefer the more cerebral or cultural environs of book clubs or theatergoing groups. Social media can provide a broad variety of opportunities for the like-minded to cross-fertilize ideas and opinions (and/or wax contentious, if that's your preferred tone, though we'd recommend steering clear of arguments, whether online or off; you're not likely to change anyone's mind, and you may well destroy your mood).

Whether you are seeking romance or just a great friend with well-developed listening skills, you'll find that others are looking for companionship just like you. One thing for sure: you won't find good company by sitting alone at home. Get enthusiastic. Own the project. If you're reasonably comfortable in a crowd, even if you're not a natural born icebreaker, you can still get out more and open yourself up to the possibility of a serendipitous encounter. You may meet someone more fabulous than you ever thought possible; or you could make the rounds to countless singles parties, cruises, and poetry readings only to find yourself nearly as lonely as you were before, albeit a bit more entertained.

If you're more the shy and retiring type, you may need to stretch those vulnerability muscles. A frank conversation with an old acquaintance can sometimes point you in the right direction, or help direct a potential new friend toward you. If such a strategy comes up short, you might just bite the bullet and join an online dating group. Some of these are sensitively administered and effective. We strongly suggest, however, that you proceed with caution; get solid references before meeting anyone in person from out of the blue. Some, not all, dating services provide references; if yours does not, it makes good sense to ask the person you're interested in for contact information for a third party who can speak for him or her. And of course spend some time emailing or conversing with a prospective date or friend before agreeing to meet somewhere public, safe, and neutral, until you have established trust.

Dating as a seasoned, well-marinated baby boomer can actually be far more gratifying and less anxiety-producing than it was back in our greener days. We can now enjoy the distinct advantage of having learned a thing or two about who we are. Especially if you've worked your way through some of the values-clarifying, roles-defining exercises we offered back in Part One, your life has become more purpose-driven and self-aware. If you are fortunate enough (or open enough) to meet Ms. or Mr. Right the second or third time around, it will more likely be with open eyes. And if you should happen to fall in love, it will be less about falling and more about ascending together to new heights, with all the ripe wisdom of maturity. Who can say that such a liaison won't prove to be a long-awaited bond with Mr. or Ms. Righter-than-ever-before?

While at first glance one might think that introverts would find it more difficult to reach out to others, we'd like to suggest that the extrovert faces his or her own challenges. The sanguine, crowd-friendly, socially adept single

CASE STUDY: US

When Simcha and I began dating, we were fifty-eight and sixty-one respectively. I was hesitant, to say the least. The last time I'd been "on the market," I was a surfer girl vying for the lifeguard's eye. Suddenly there was something unsettling about looking in the mirror. Moreover, the two of us represented the classic extrovert/introvert dichotomy.

We figured it out, though, partly with the help of this quote from Antoine de Saint-Exupéry, author of The Little Prince: *"Love does not consist of gazing at each other, but in looking outward together in the same direction."*

—Frumma

tends to be defined by relationships with others more than by an inner sense of self. That can have its advantages—the introvert can easily cross the line and become pathologically self-absorbed—but extroversion can also be a trap. One can forfeit one's own preferences and sense of personal identity in favor of what makes the group a group. Optimally, the mature approach to social interaction calls for a fine blend of quiet, focused, inner awareness and the ability to lose oneself and have fun with others.

How, then, does the extrovert get in touch with his or her inner introvert, and vice versa? You may find this strangely counterintuitive, but we think there's a single answer to both challenges.

"To Thine Own Self Be True?"

Well, no, that's not quite it. But it's close.

This famous phrase was uttered not by some wise champion of self-actualization, but by Polonius, a rather clueless pedant in *Hamlet,* whose character Shakespeare probably meant to portray as epitomizing bad advice. Focusing on yourself is not likely to be the best way to win friends and influence people. Nor is it likely to lead you to actual truth.

But paradoxically, if we can go a little deeper than our own obvious preferences and perspectives, we might just come to recognize a more essential self—a self that can help the shy loner get over himself *and* assist the social butterfly in becoming more internally grounded and real. Because the true essence of who we all are, by virtue of our innermost souls, is not limited to either introversion or extroversion. What drives us when we are at our best is not our various quirks of personality. The genuine self to whom we want to be true—if we want to be *getting better all the time*—is not some artificial construct of self-image. Who are we really?

We are givers.

We've all heard the Beatles sing, "The love you take is equal to the love you make." But have we taken that astute observation to heart? Or are we still waiting passively for love to find us? We may think we've learned Dale Carnegie's secret key to getting others interested in us, but are we actively pursuing our interest in *them*? Or are we still just feeling entitled to someone else's attention?

Reflect on a time when you were especially happy. More than likely it involved your bestowing benevolence on another—a child, a student, a parent, a lover. Love overcomes loneliness; giving love evokes stronger feelings than receiving love.

Think of ways you can give, and keep giving, without overthinking whether you have what to give. Help a friend make a tough decision; bring dinner to your overwhelmed daughter-in-law; invite a new acquaintance for a cup of tea; pick up the phone and call someone you know who is depressed or ailing. Fix your widowed neighbor's flapping shutter or shovel her walk after a storm. Make sure your jumper cables are handy so you can help people on the side of the road.

. . . .

MUST IT ALL BE RANDOM?

The campaign to carry out random acts of kindness, admirably promoted by such diverse celebrities as Princess Diana, the Dalai Lama, and Lady Gaga, has grown increasingly popular ever since author Anne Herbert first scribbled the phrase on a restaurant placemat back in 1983.

We'd just like to point out our belief that at its core, kindness is not random; it is intentional—and the more intentional and deliberate our acts of kindness, the less random this world will become. King David wrote, "The world is built with loving kindness." Let us define and refine our good intentions and help rebuild this often haphazard world in the image of that original benevolence.

. . . .

Be creative, be loving, be audacious. Why not send an unsolicited care package to a close friend or family member, just because? Take time and care to put thoughtful items in it; make things rather than buy them. Have as much fun with the packaging as with its contents. Infuse the package with your loving thoughts, and imagine how pleased (and/or surprised) they'll be when they receive it.

"Service," said someone long forgotten, before the line was canonized by Muhammad Ali, "is the rent we pay for the privilege of taking up space in this world." We'd like to suggest that service is actually a far more powerful investment than the mere paying of rent. It renders us owners, not renters; it transforms us from residents into architects. Every act of kindness we perform reaches deep into the best of us and extends that precious essence outward toward the world. If that's not an antidote to loneliness, we don't know what is.

Professor Shawn Achor of Harvard, a prominent advocate of keeping a daily gratitude notebook (see chapter 6), includes one daily act of kindness in his prescription for happiness. It's a good place to start, and can lead to a quality of life wherein service becomes not just our *raison d'être*, but the vehicle that brings love and companionship into our lives. According to David R. Hamilton, PhD, author of *Why Kindness Is Good for You*, kindness makes us happier because when we do something nice for someone else, we feel good about who we are.[35] On a biochemical level, acts of kindness activate what's been called a "helper's high," elevating our internal levels of endorphins, the brain's natural mood enhancers.

Without getting too technical, here's a quick look at the cascade of positive events that takes place when an act of kindness triggers an upsurge of psychoneuroimmunological well-being. In concert with the wave of emotional warmth, levels of dopamine and oxytocin increase throughout the body, especially in the brain. Among other benefits, this is particularly advantageous for heart health. Oxytocin, known as a cardioprotective hormone, triggers the release of nitric oxide, which expands the blood vessels and thus reduces blood pressure. Oxytocin also reduces the levels of free radicals and inflammation in the cardiovascular system—major contributors to the aging process.

Dr. Hamilton also points to research that shows a relationship between compassion and the vagus nerve, one of the cranial nerves. Among other functions, this nerve regulates inflammation in the body, affecting what is known as the *inflammatory reflex*. Inflammation is a major contributor to all types of disease. Therefore, through acts of kindness, aging, as well as heart disease, is slowed at its source.

Needless to say, kindness is good for the world at large. What can we possibly do as individuals to counteract the violence and lack of empathy that characterize the world around us? Daily reports of senseless brutality and terrorism shake us to our core. Our default response is often a feeling of helplessness. When we're kind, we inspire others to be kind, thereby creating a ripple effect that spreads outwards. As a pebble creates ripples when dropped in a pond, acts of kindness radiate outwards, touching others' lives, propagating benevolence everywhere, until the ripple becomes a tidal wave that cycles back and lifts our own boats along with those of others.

. . . .

OPPORTUNITIES ABOUND

Looking for places to give of yourself? An online search for community service reveals hundreds of possibilities, from tutoring and home health volunteering to safe driving assistance and helping people file their taxes. As our search expanded, we uncovered a wealth of potential adventures for those with the time and the guts to let go of whatever vine they've been swinging on till now, including these:

Tourism Cares (www.tourismcares.org) offers ways for volunteers to help protect and restore national parks, botanical gardens, and other travel destinations across the country.

You might find fulfillment as a sports coach, counselor, or instructor through the American Camp Association (www.acacamps.org). At some camps, you can even teach kids to become volunteers.

Fly for Good Network (www.flyforgood.com) gives deep discounts on airfares to those willing to volunteer in such exotic spots as Vietnam, Ecuador, Nigeria, or Peru.

Wildlife Friends Foundation (www.wfft.org) rescues, rehabilitates, and cares for suffering wildlife in such endangered habitats as Thailand and Southeast Asia.

Created during John F. Kennedy's presidency, the overseas Peace Corps (www.peacecorps.gov) has a special portal for volunteers over the age of fifty. Recently, volunteers sixty and older have more than doubled. And the Senior

Corps (www.nationalservice.gov/programs/senior-corps) links today's fifty-five-plus population with the people and groups that need them most, contributing their skills, knowledge, and experience as mentors, coaches or companions to individuals, nonprofits, faith-based and other community organizations.

Creativity: Solitude and Society Intertwined

Charitable deeds, random or otherwise, are wonderful, but not necessarily the only expression of what it means to be a giver. Each of us is blessed with a unique gift. To discover and bestow that gift upon the world is a huge part, perhaps the truest part, of why we are here. Though we sometimes feel alone, we are seamlessly connected to a world that is waiting for us to emerge with the uniqueness we are meant to bring.

Being single at sixty-something is an exercise in discovering our singularity, our individuality, even for those of us who are blessed with loving relationships. It's necessary to bravely step into the aloneness from time to time, to unearth those hidden gifts, so that we can then step back out and paint that masterpiece or sing that song—optimally, in harmony with a kindred soul or souls.

One marvelous tool we've discovered to unleash the creativity within is Julia Cameron's book *The Artist's Way*.[36] It's not just for artists. It's a practical guide to getting in touch with your own internal voice, a way of becoming your own closest companion. As such, it becomes a springboard for unblocking the giving of your gift—be it in writing, creating music, some other expression of your talents, or simply in communicating freely and openly with the people who share your world.

Workshops available on the Internet or in your community can help you get started; or you can explore the Artist's Way on your own. Cameron's program consists primarily of introducing two practices into your life—one daily and one weekly.

The daily practice is called *morning pages*. Immediately upon rising in the morning, we take pen to paper and write three pages of longhand, stream-of-consciousness, unfiltered monologue. The pages aren't meant to be planned, edited, or even reread; they're a means of siphoning off the mind's surface noise and achieving flow so that we can access and exercise our deeper thoughts and impulses. Cameron describes morning pages as metabolizing life. Sometimes the process helps us to work through painful or intense passages, such as death, divorce, or loss of a friend. In a more upbeat mode, the pages can act as a muse or a cheerleader, spurring us on to dream new dreams or enthusiastically take that next step. Or they can serve as an early warning system, allowing us to attend to some intuitive sense that something is amiss.

The cumulative effect of daily morning pages is extraordinary. We grow more intimate with ourselves and, as a result, more intimately engaged with the world outside ourselves.

The weekly practice is the *artist's date*—a solitary excursion to a location that has the potential to inspire or excite you or pique your creative interest in something new. It could be a thrift shop or museum or bookstore, a botanical garden or some mysterious, ethnic culinary outlet.

Cameron notes that while morning pages are work, the artist's date is play—which actually makes it more challenging for many people to do. Playfulness, whimsy, imagination, even mischief, are among the characteristics of youth that we would be wise to reclaim as we advance in age.

We are too wise, and we've come too far, to just let things happen. We can be the force that transforms empty, lonely days into Third Acts permeated with purpose and passion. The project we didn't make time for when we were thirty-something, the song fragment we didn't finish writing because there were more pressing concerns, are still there on our back burners. We can check off items on our bucket lists and travel to exotic locales or tend to our own home gardens, however small, just to feel new life sprouting between our fingers. We can awaken with the sunrise, walk along unfamiliar trails, and watch how life unfolds out where nature is unashamed. When we rekindle our fascination with society's high roads and back alleys, we inevitably become more alluring and attractive to the fellow travelers we will encounter along the way.

We have a friend who brews kombucha, a fermented, effervescent tea-based drink whose probiotic properties are purported to have amazing health benefits. As with wine-making, it takes time for the elixir to ripen and mature. It's a private, almost meditative enterprise that entails riding

the slow tide of time, patiently awaiting the graceful evolution of biochemical change. She allows herself to notice the
pace of transformation, and puts it to work.

That same active appreciation of time's inexorable
advance is a key component in allowing our inner awareness, acquired in solitude, to blossom into qualitative
change in our social lives. Embracing both the aloneness
and the oneness with others, we can grow whole.

Whole also implies *wholesome*, as we shall see presently
in the next chapter on that most indispensable form of
wealth: health.

❧ 14 ❧

To Your Good Health

We don't stop playing because we grow old.
We grow old because we stop playing.
—GEORGE BERNARD SHAW

As the 1960s came crashing to a close, a group of kindred souls converged on a rented farmhouse not far from a university campus in upstate New York. It was a homecoming of sorts. Most had either graduated from or dropped out of this school some years earlier. After various adventures around the world, alive and kicking, though somewhat worse for wear, they were there to regroup and recoup their squandered sense of themselves.

This motley crew shared one thing in common—a passion for homegrown food and a healthy lifestyle. A half-acre organic garden and a few hundred-pound sacks of whole grains provided breakfast, lunch, and dinner for the core group of friends and numerous drop-in guests. They read books on nutrition and cooking and planetary wellness, studied with mentors about meditation and exercise, and chewed their food carefully and consciously as a gateway to harmony with the order of the universe.

It wasn't a cult. There was no leader, just a fortuitous gathering of independent seekers who before long went their separate ways again. Some stayed in touch. Two of them partnered up and opened a health food restaurant the following year. Their customers—mostly a college crowd—used to say that the bowls of miso soup and brown rice and veggies got them high. Whatever; they were young and impressionable, and those were heady times.

The partners called the restaurant Belly of the Whale. Like the biblical Jonah, who was swallowed by a big fish, they found temporary respite there from challenges they weren't quite willing to face. After a couple of years they were ready to move on, having gained from the experience an emerging sense of how biological health can open a door to spiritual awakening. One of those partners was Simcha, your humble coauthor.

Around the same time, Frumma was investing time and energy as a pioneering entrepreneur, running a chain of natural food emporiums in Colorado. She was also giving cooking classes and serving on the start-up Board of Organic Merchants. This was the beginning of what eventually grew into the Great American Health Food Movement.

It would be few decades before tofu and coconut oil would be available on the shelves of your local supermarket. In those days it was counterculture, if not revolutionary. When the Beatles sang, "You know that what you eat you are," it was big news. And although it purported to be all

FRUMMA'S BIG BREAK

One brisk morning in 1969, an enterprising young space cadet who worked in our health food store in Boulder asked if we'd be interested in investing in his herb tea startup. He and his partner had gotten into collecting wild herbs in the nearby mountains and packaging innovative blends. We loaned Mo Siegel $5,000 to help get the business off to a good start. About six months later, his sales growing rapidly, Mo offered us a choice: he could repay the loan or make us partners in the enterprise. I decided the whole operation was a tad on the flaky side and chose repayment. The rest is history—as in his story, not mine. Celestial Seasonings Teas made many millions, and is today a giant, expanding health food conglomerate.

My story (and I'm sticking to it) is that despite the wealth that coulda/shoulda/woulda been mine, I am convinced that had I made the more astute financial choice at the time, I'd have missed out on the personal riches, the spiritual rewards, and the undeniable delights of my journey through life.

The smart money is always on true destiny.

about diet and physical health, it had unmistakable spiritual overtones as well. People were starting to understand that the body and the mind are inextricably intertwined, not separate parts of us, and that physical health is a function of factors beyond biology.

New "revolutionary" diets seem to appear every year. People are easily confused by too much information or advice that comes from unreliable sources with question-able agendas. It isn't easy to distinguish the facts from the fads. Sometimes even traditional knowledge bases and common sense can be clouded by quasi-spiritual New Age hype and hoopla.

Scientific studies can also be poorly designed or taken out of context. Questions should always be asked of any study: Where is the data coming from, and how was it obtained? Is it reputable research, or advocacy in the service of commerce, whether by the dairy council, the nutraceu-tical supplement industry, the cattlemen's beef association, or the American Medical Association?

Who can say which diet is best for me: plant-based, paleo, Mediterranean, high-carb-low-fat, gluten-free, raw vegan? By the time you're reading this book, half of today's diets may be outdated and the experts will be debating some new nutritional theory.

And that's just the food part. What about other factors that affect health?

We've spent the better part of our adult lives and careers sorting out the sound principles of a healthy life-style and guiding people in applying them. As important as preventative medical strategies are at any age, they are all the more essential for people over sixty, who are particu-larly vulnerable to chronic or catastrophic illness. We keep abreast of modern, ongoing research, which strongly sug-gests that a combination of diet, exercise, stress reduction, and proper sleep can prevent or reverse disease.

Our perspective is also rooted in teachings that have evolved out of the ancient wisdom traditions of East and West. Many of our sources go back thousands of years, such as the annals of Chinese and East Asian medicine, or over many centuries, as with the medical writings of Moses Maimonides. When we offer advice, it is based not only on recent studies and our own personal and clinical experience, but on a vast literature of case histories, theory, and empirical observation.

Nonetheless, we don't often presume to tell people what they ought to do. Even when asked to prescribe a nutritional regimen, we generally prefer to convey the principles and let people make their own choices. Like nature itself, every human being is an unfathomable mystery. There is no one-size-fits-all path to health and well-being. Even the great physician-scholars of history, some of whom were able to proclaim with great certainty the most life-supporting ways of living, would humbly acknowledge the limits of their own wisdom. So we do the best we can, and pray for illumination from the unknowable Source of our knowing.

All that said, here's a brief compendium of our most basic, tried-and-true principles, offered in the hope that with the help of these guidelines you'll keep getting better all the time, for a long time to come.

We break it down into three useful compartments: nutrition, exercise, and attitude. They do overlap, but then so does everything.

Nutrition: You Are What You Eat . . .
Also What You Don't

Simply put, *metabolism* is a fancy word for turning food into energy. On a slightly deeper level, it's about turning parts of the world that aren't yet you into you. You don't have to be a gourmet or gourmand to appreciate that food is profoundly important to your health and well-being.

Here's the cycle of transformation in a nutshell. Vegetables absorb mineral substances so that they can *grow*. Animals consume minerals too, but add vegetables to the regimen not just to grow, but to be able to *move* independently. They also *emote*. (Some animals eat other animals; their emotions are that much more fierce.) Humans eat all three—minerals, vegetables, and animals—and raise the stakes of the game considerably: we don't only grow, move, and feel; we *think*, and *speak*, and organize societies, ideally with an evolving sense of higher purpose.

So it's not merely energy that we acquire from what we eat; it's also quality of life. As such, nutrition is more than just a numbers game. Counting calories, meeting the recommended daily allowances of nutrients, or totaling up grams of fat and salt and sugar doesn't necessary tell us what we need to know about eating well. In fact, this sort of quantitative analysis can be part of the problem because it can obscure one of the most significant principles of proper nourishment, as we age: *less is more.*

Most research supports the fact that as we get older, we need less food. Truth be told, most of us, including younger people, live a lifestyle characterized more by too much food than too little. We who live amidst unprecedented abundance are so accustomed to overindulging that we've nearly forgotten what real appetite is. Food has become entertainment, distraction, addiction, or antidepressant. The part of the brain that neuro-science calls the *satiety center*, which tells us when we've had enough to eat, acts like it's blown a fuse. As a result, instead of injecting vitality and stoking the fires of enthusiastic and joyful activity, eating brings us down.

THREE-QUARTERS FULL RULE

Fortunately there's a rule of thumb that is ridiculously simple (though it can be challenging to master; as we've mentioned, bad habits die hard.) Are you ready for this?

Eat only when hungry. Never fill yourself completely. *Stop eating when three-quarters full.*

Many people to whom we offer this advice (and, we must confess, sometimes we ourselves) discover that it's difficult to know when you are three-quarters full. So when in doubt, err on the side of emptiness and wait fifteen minutes. We promise you that when you find yourself genuinely hungry again, food will not have gone out of style.

This may be your single most important key to good health. You are leaving room not just for good digestion, which turns food efficiently into energy rather than fat, but also for vigorous circulation of all the enzymes, hormones, blood cells, bodily fluids, clear thinking, and positive emotion that will keep you gloriously and vivaciously alive and well. In a very real sense, you are making room for miracles.

Is it really that simple? Yes and no. Other principles assist this one in working its magic, but this is rule number one, and it makes the others easier as well. It is mostly a preventive strategy rather than a therapeutic diet, so those of us with existing problems may require more specific consultation with an expert who understands the healing arts as well as dietary guidelines.

OTHER NUTRITION TIPS

Here's a short list of additional suggestions. They're not the entire story, but they will aid your quest for vibrant health and wellness.

- ❧ Start each day with fresh-squeezed lemon juice and raw honey, stirred into a cup of hot water, first thing in the morning, and only on an empty stomach. If you make only one change to your daily regimen, make it this one! It's practically effortless, yet its benefits are extraordinary. It will augment energy and reduce stress; facilitate improved metabolism and weight loss; balance your blood chemistry and reduce inflammation; prevent constipation and improve colon function; cleanse and flush the urinary and biliary tracts; clear the body of phlegmy accumulation; and promote oral hygiene and radiant skin. And it's delicious! We recommend the juice of approximately half a lemon and a teaspoon of raw honey, or more, to taste. You will be able to digest it quickly; you can follow up ten or fifteen minutes later with your preferred breakfast.

- If you enjoy (or depend on) caffeine in the morning, try adding a teabag to the lemon-honey mix. It'll give you the needed boost, and help you cut down on or eliminate coffee, which for many of us has a not-so-beneficial effect on blood chemistry.

∽ Balanced meals (and an overall balanced diet) are a key to good health. But *balance* can be defined in many different and confusing ways. Acid or alkaline? Carbs or proteins? Insulin or glucagon? Yin or yang? Government-recommended food pyramids that change radically every few years? Again, don't obsess over quantitative rules. Try these simple strategies, find a method that works for you, and the more complex details of balance will take care of themselves:

- If your diet includes animal protein, a good rule of thumb is to visualize your plate divided in thirds, with one-third for protein and the other two-thirds for plant based-foods—whole grains, cooked vegetables, and salads.

- Pay attention to creating a colorful presentation on the plate. Select a menu with variety of colors. Don't let everything at the table be all brown, or all white, or even all green. This may seem superficial, but you'll be surprised at how nutritionally meaningful it can become.

- Still more significantly, a variety of flavors can also ensure a balanced regimen. The basic tastes are sweet, spicy, sour, bitter, bland, and salty. According to traditional medicine, each taste stimulates a different internal organ system. Meals that artfully combine the various tastes—balancing your personal preferences with complementary flavors—will keep your internal organs talking to one another.

- ❧ Cooked vegetables (not overcooked!) are generally more beneficial for digestion than raw. Cold and raw foods tend to make the metabolism sluggish and slow. Similarly, avoid iced drinks. Warm beverages and room-temperature water are best. Try not to drink a lot with meals; chew well rather than washing your food down. (This preference for cooked meals is somewhat controversial, as many vegetarians and raw-foods enthusiasts disagree. In fact, a short-term raw diet can have a cleansing, therapeutic effect, but for most of us, especially in cooler climates and among the elderly or infirm, a raw diet is not a sustainable way of life in the long run. Moderate amounts of salads are fine.)

- ❧ Don't be afraid of carbs. Brown rice and chocolate brownies are both carbohydrates, but they are worlds apart in their effects on your body and blood sugar. Similarly, don't fear fats; your body needs them. Just avoid trans fats and choose healthy oils, such as extra virgin olive oil, coconut oil, and grapeseed oil. High-quality essential fatty acids are also found in such foods as salmon, avocados, nuts, and seeds.

ᴝ Eat seated at the table, never standing up. Try not to multitask while eating; keep cell phones and reading materials away from the table. Such distractions lead to overeating and feeling unfulfilled. Approach your food in a calm and grateful mood.

. . . .

MORE HELPFUL HINTS

- *Avoid white sugar, artificial sweeteners, colorings, and MSG.*
- *Use sea salt or Himalayan pink salt rather than refined table salt.*
- *Make changes gradually. Radical changes in diet can trigger illness.*
- *Stay away from processed foods with long lists of artificial ingredients. Choose simple, whole foods.*
- *Eat fruits in moderation, and only alone, never with or immediately after meals. This applies especially to fruit juices.*
- *For weight loss, try to minimize milled flour products like breads, pasta, or pastries.*
- *Many people have issues with wheat. It's only rarely about gluten, and the jury is out as to the dangers of GMO (genetically modified) foods. The biggest offenders are the pesticides. Choose organically grown wheat products whenever you can, and you will feel better.*
- *Heal and enrich gut health with probiotic foods, such as live yogurt, naturally fermented sauerkraut, miso, and kombucha—especially if you have taken antibiotics.*

- *Fortify core energies and immunity with bone broths,
  such as organic chicken soup or soup stock made with
  bones of grass-fed beef and lamb.*
- *Avoid the microwave; use stainless steel, ceramic,
  and glassware rather than aluminum and nonstick
  cookware.*

Exercise: Poetry in Motion

The second essential in self-care is exercise. A host of studies has shown that exercise helps promote a healthier and longer life. People over age sixty with better cardio-respiratory fitness appear to live longer than unfit adults, regardless of their levels of body fat. A five-year study published in the *Journal of the American Medical Association* even found that people who exercised and followed a healthy diet diminished their risk of Alzheimer's by as much as 60 percent.[37] From muscle cells to blood cells to brain cells, it don't mean a thing if it ain't got that zing.

What sort of exercise is best? How do we get started if we're a little late to the party or need to improve our current routine? What's the motivation and perspective that will get us up off the couch and keep us moving?

Movement equals life. Contemplate the movement of the universe: it grows, sways, shifts, rotates, orbits, breathes, flexes, extends, clenches, and releases its way into all its relationships. We may not always be in perfect harmony with the music of the celestial spheres, but if we listen well, we can dance to its beat. Nature is the best personal trainer.

In today's urbanized, alienating world, most of us suffer from a nature deficiency. We are surrounded by concrete, oblivious to the rhythms of life, imprisoned in mazes of straight lines and right angles. No wonder we don't know how to move. Or when we do, it's with a stiff and rigid creakiness or jerkiness that hurts more than it helps. We need to get out in nature more often—take a hike or a walk, or simply look up and watch the clouds in the sky go by. In Japan, they have a term for it: *forest bathing*. One of the preeminent professors at Tokyo's Nippon Medical School has studied its effects. He found that in addition to reducing feelings of stress, anxiety, or anger, simply spending a few calm, contemplative hours in natural surroundings can increase energy and immunity.[38]

By extension, we can learn to model our intentional exercise programs on the natural movements of wind and water, clouds and planets, flora and fauna. What, your local gym doesn't offer a class on imitating the solar system? No worries. We can avail ourselves of more conventional exercise opportunities while keeping this somewhat lyrical approach in mind.

Exercise can be divided into four basic types: *aerobic exercise*, *flexibility training*, *strength training*, and the *cultivation of balance*. Though specific routines are beyond the scope of this book, let's take a brief look at the basic elements of each type.

∽ **Aerobic exercise** stimulates lung function, brings color to the face, and helps the heart pump oxygen to the organs and muscles. For many of us, a daily brisk walk is preferable to running, because it is low-impact and therefore unlikely to result in injury. Similarly, swimming and biking are excellent forms of exercise; other options include tennis, Zumba or other dance forms, step aerobics, and the like. The ideal guideline is thirty minutes of aerobic exercise daily, if you can, or at least several times a week. If a half-hour is too much for your schedule or your stamina, try ten-minute workouts. Many begin by keeping track of their steps each day with an electronic step counter. A good goal is to walk ten thousand steps per day.

Interestingly (here's an example of where exercise and dietary advice overlap), the great physician Moses Maimonides said that to promote good digestion and efficient metabolism, one shouldn't sit down to a meal before exercising enough to redden the face and break a sweat.

Aerobics will boost the size of your brain and improve working memory, planning, multitasking, and other cognitive functions. It also lowers blood sugar and triglycerides, improves cardiac fitness, and reduces the risk of cancer. What you may notice most of all is the way exercise produces endorphins—feel-good neuropeptides that chase the blues away much more effectively and safely than antidepressants.

ॐ **Flexibility training** also benefits both the body and the spirit, though in a different way. It's slower, calmer, and more conducive to a contemplative or meditative experience. On the physical, musculoskeletal level, stretching exercises or postural adjustments can prevent or relieve aches and pains and keep muscles and tendons long and limber. In addition, they can help induce a more supple and resilient state of mind.

Frumma attends two yoga classes a week and has been doing so on and off for many years. Though its origins are often associated with Indian and Hindu culture, yoga has evolved into a culturally neutral practice with which Westerners can be comfortable. Many of the same or similar principles of movement, posture, and breath can also be found in Pilates and Feldenkrais training. Done correctly, under the tutelage of an astute teacher, yoga can be one of the most effective forms of mindful stretching and flexibility training. Unfortunately, in our opinion some of the modern iterations of "power yoga" have become overly forceful or competitive. So be careful, go slowly, and listen to your own body as you proceed. Some will do best with a gentle, easygoing "restorative" yoga class.

Another option (and this is Simcha's preference) is the practice of *qigong* (pronounced "chee-gong"), a form of cultivating subtle internal energies, harmonious breathing, and musculoskeletal wellness that originated in China. It's been described as the therapeutic or medical aspect of the Chinese martial arts, such as *Tai Ji Quan* (sometimes called *Tai Chi*) or *Gong Fu* (*Kung Fu*). Qigong has remarkable healing and consciousness-raising qualities that can free up inner resources of energy, alertness, and confidence we never imagined we had. It's also a perfect complement to forest bathing or other experiences in natural surroundings. There's nothing quite like twenty or thirty minutes of qigong on the beach.

We're often unaware of how much tension we hold in our bodies and how that exacerbates stress—the root of many diseases. Gentle forms of flexibility training help us to release unwelcome stress. Just as aerobic exercise pumps up the flow of oxygen in our lungs, stretching oxygenates the brain while relaxing the mind and the body. This training reduces stress in a manner similar to meditation and mindfulness practices (see chapter 5).

Once learned, these principles of harmonious movement, mindful breathing, and good posture can be applied even in the midst of casual everyday activities. Once acquired, the skill of simply shifting the attention from external stress to inner ease will bring you incalculable rewards.

❧ **Strength training** and calisthenics are more conventional forms of exercise, and they too can be an important component of an Age Well Now fitness program. Working with light weights or resistance-training machines in mildly challenging settings will improve not only muscular mass and joint mobility, but bone density as well. It can also be crucial to regulating glucose metabolism, reducing belly fat, and preventing diabetes and heart disease. Just don't pump iron with such intensity as to hurt yourself. Many repetitions with small weights are better than trying to emulate some young muscle-bound body builder using free weights or heavy-duty Nautilus machines. Bicep curls, reverse curls, tricep extensions, modified squats, lunges, and push-ups are all great in moderation. Ten to fifteen minutes per session is plenty. Be sure to leave a little recovery time (a couple of days between sessions) to give your muscles a chance to rest and bounce back. Always stretch slowly and easily before and after a workout. (And don't forget about those Kegels we mentioned back in chapter 10.)

If you're prone to low-back pain or sciatica, core training of the abdominal torso area is key, with an emphasis on crunches rather than full sit-ups. When doing crunches, remember to look at the ceiling and support your head so you don't strain your neck. Start with perhaps ten reps a day, and build from there. We also recommend working with a big, bright-colored Pilates ball. It's more fun than crunching on the floor—and the grandchildren will love it too!

ﾍ **Balance training** is the last but certainly not least important form of essential exercise. As with a balanced diet, the idea of balance can mean different things to different people. Here we're referring to the simple physical practice of standing steadily, either on one foot at a time or while doing knee bends and toe lifts, without leaning on anything or falling down. Many older people begin to lose their ability to balance, which can result in the all-too-common tendency to fall and break bones. A hip fracture often triggers a downward spiral in other aspects of health, heaven forfend.

Two or three minutes of balance exercise a day makes a huge difference. Many of the popular yoga poses or qigong forms emphasize balance. If you prefer, however, you can keep it simple and informal. Just try standing on one leg while lifting the other leg, breathing from the lower abdomen, and gazing at a fixed point on the wall in front of you. If you can only hold this pose for a few seconds, fine—don't give up! Soon it will be twenty, then thirty, then sixty seconds or more.

You can also surreptitiously stand on one leg while you are waiting in line at the supermarket; start by holding on to the shopping cart and then letting go. Or stand on your tiptoes while doing the dishes.

Before long, balance exercises will be about more than just physical balance. They will help you develop balance in other ways as well, such as gaining a sense of inner poise, trust, mental clarity, and emotional equilibrium.

One great benefit of a balanced approach to life is the ability to resolve apparent conflicts, to see both sides of an issue and consider opposing points of view from a broader, more inclusive perspective. This is significant not just in mediating effectively between antagonists, but in harmonizing inner conflict as well. For example, how often do we find ourselves torn between an individualistic drive toward personal fulfillment and the demands of family or community that call for selfless devotion and sacrifice? We are each unique, yet we are all oarsmen in one boat.

IN THE STILL OF THE NIGHT

A still deeper quality of equilibrium is reached through balance between the active aspects of our lives and the quiet state of being we achieve when we allow ourselves to rest. This is the dance of *do-be-do-be-do* we explored back in chapter 3. It establishes a finely tuned balance between willful activity, on the one hand, and the quietude that connects us with who we truly are. We gain two distinct benefits: this balance nourishes an internal sense of confidence and calm, and it awakens the energy we need to succeed.

Sleep is another key component of a healthy, balanced lifestyle. Old habits left over from our hyperactive, workaholic Second Acts leave many of us Third Actors unnecessarily sleep-deprived. Make sufficient sleep one of your nightly rituals. Select a good mattress, especially if you're susceptible to low-back pain. And remember the proverbial, incontrovertible, old-school wisdom of early-to-bed regularity. We each have different needs; our sleep patterns change as we get older. After a comprehensive two-year study, the National Sleep Foundation recommends a steady regimen of seven to eight hours of sleep every night for older adults.[39] Your mileage may vary.

Attitude: A Good Eye, A Good Heart

The English word *health* is derived from the Old English *haelth*, which means *wholth* (OK, not an actual word) or *wholeness*. The reason? Genuine health is not a piecemeal endeavor. Longevity is like hitting a home run: you've got to come full circle and touch all the bases on the way. As we've pointed out, *all the bases* means the physical, emotional, intellectual, and spiritual dimensions of our lives.

Except that life is not baseball. It's not really a game at all, except insofar as we have fun living it. No one clever metaphor will suffice to shed light on what we really want to say here. But let's try this: life is a celebration. Whether we are focusing at any given moment on our bodies, minds, hearts, or souls, the way to wholeness—the key to having all our parts sing in four-part harmony—is to do so with *joy*.

One small example: we are often called upon to advise people who want to lose weight, feel better, have more energy, or come unstuck from their dysfunctional relationships with food. No two people are the same, so each individual will usually need some sort of customized assistance. A common thread, however, invariably makes its way into our conversations. The two worst things you can do with your diet, we tell them, is to eat foods you don't like because you think they're good for you, or to eat things you love but believe are bad for you. Either way, you're living in the middle of a disconnect. As a result, your metabolism inevitably breaks down. You need to be wholly enthused and aligned with yourself or else become your own worst enemy. Yes, be smart and selective, but make sure your prudent food choices are as delightful as they are healthful. Lighten up, and bon appétit—enjoy!

Attitude of gratitude has become a cliché (and we've no doubt bludgeoned you enough with its importance in previous chapters), but it's nonetheless the way to be well. To be appreciative and grateful for every blessing—especially the blessings about which we haven't yet figured out *how* they're blessings—is to live life with a good eye. A good eye tries to see the good in everything and everyone.

A good eye leads to a good heart. A spirit of generosity toward others, a kind word, a charitable deed—all these are also acts of kindness toward oneself. They nurture the sort of wellness that no medicine can provide, no nutrients can feed: it's the wellness that lies within the very essence of who we are. And it happens to be the closest thing to a guarantee that we'll stay happy. To paraphrase the wise King Solomon in Proverbs 15:15, "A person with a good heart celebrates nonstop."

In Simcha's acupuncture clinic, there's a sign on the wall that reminds him and his patients of a classical Chinese medical aphorism. It reads, *bu tong ze tong; tong ze bu tong*, which means, *where there is openness, there is no pain; where there is pain, there is obstruction.* Free-flowing openness is the secret to well-being. Blockage is the path to agony. In purely physical terms, the saying is about promoting efficient circulation and removing internal obstacles, whether in the form of muscular rigidity, stagnant digestive processes, or emotional stress. But the openness that is synonymous with health and wellness is more than simply physical.

In a sense, to be open and flowing freely is to be connected, both internally and externally. We've spoken about effective, congruent communication between the mind and the heart. We've emphasized the importance of staying aligned with a purpose, a mission in life. We've shared experience and insights as to how to cultivate quality relationships with loved ones and not-so-loved ones.

Most of all, we urge everyone to remain in touch with spiritual source, however we understand that; and perhaps even more so, in ways that are beyond our understanding. Embedded within every one of the healthy strategies we've touched upon in this chapter there is an unseen spiritual dimension. Even in the most physical, down-to-earth exercises, like weight lifting and crunches and chewing your food well, there's a *meta*physical aspect that makes it all work. It's present and available when we need it, and—most significantly—when we allow it into our lives.

Case in point: a few years ago Simcha was suddenly knocked for a loop with an excruciating case of low-back pain, most likely the result of a ridiculously ill-advised all-night/all-day solo drive of about 1500 miles. Neither his acupuncturist colleagues nor a friend who happens to be one of the most gifted chiropractors in town nor 800 milligrams of ibuprofen could help. It took a lot of rest, stretching, breathing meditation, massage, and an anti-inflammatory diet to get him back on his feet. But still, days later, the pain and frustration were intense enough to motivate a nearly desperate midnight prayer for relief. Something remarkable then happened. Reaching out—or rather, reaching *inward*—to the presence of a higher source of healing, Simcha experienced a direct connection to that often elusive source. The painful obstruction gave way instantly to a feeling of release, out of nowhere, bringing a flow of warmth to muscle and bone. Just like that, the ordeal was over.

The so-called barriers between our bodies, our minds, and our souls are not as real as we think they are. Perception may be limited, but life is infinite. And it's possible (not always easy, perhaps, but possible!) to remember and connect with that sense of boundless vitality in every move we make.

A friend of ours in the insurance business told us just the other day about a phone conversation he had with a potential client who is well over ninety years of age. It seemed the gentleman could not find a free moment to meet. Our friend, exasperated, asked this ninety-year-old what on earth could keep him so busy. He replied that he works two shifts every day in the post office, leaves home at the crack of dawn, and doesn't get home till 11 p.m. He has followed this same routine for decades.

"Why do you feel you have to work so hard?" our astonished friend inquired.

"Because I once read that a body in motion tends to stay in motion."

As a simple man, the fellow may or may not have known that this is a phrase taken from Newton's first law of inertia. But he was clearly in touch with a higher law. Call it the law of perpetual purpose. Want a life that's whole, hale, and hearty? Remember where you're coming from; have some idea of where you're going, and why; and with that in mind, keep moving.

✒ 15 ✒

On the Ropes, Out of the Woods

Whatever doesn't kill you makes you stronger.
—FRIEDRICH NIETZSCHE

It was a warm February in the heart of Florida's horse country. A couple of dozen adventurous women of diverse backgrounds gathered from all over America for a soul-searching retreat, taking up residence in the rustic, double-decker bunks of a children's summer camp.

Around campfires till the wee hours, they shared stories of life's challenges. Along hiking trails, they saw symbolic guideposts for personal transformation in untamed, over-grown nature. On yoga mats in the meadows, in a dining hall graced with broccoli sprouts and raw kale, they toned up and trimmed down. Everyone felt 200 percent lighter, if not enlightened.

Frumma was there as a coach and presenter as well as a participant. On the last day of the retreat everyone signed on—some with a bit of trepidation—for a ropes-climbing course, a wonderful hands-on experience to hone team-building skills and grow self-esteem. Frumma saw it as a personal opportunity to learn how to better surrender her flair for leadership to the synergy of the team.

The course instructor, Clay, was a charismatic blend of a philosopher and a jock. As everyone suited up for a climb up a forty-foot pole, he said something unforgettable. "Pay careful attention to your thoughts," he told us, "and to the way you interact on the course. Because the way you do one thing is the way you'll do everything."

What had at first promised to be a fun afternoon took on new significance. It became a tool for self-knowledge, a mini-life lesson with ropes and carabiners, a bite-sized chunk of real life that was compact enough to dissect and analyze as a guide to a better future.

About six weeks later, with all the ladies back home and back in the saddle (or so they thought), something earthshaking reared its ugly head: a viral outbreak that soon became a global pandemic. It changed everything, everywhere. The repercussions of the event may or may not remain as historically devastating as they seem at this writing, while we're still in the midst of it. Time will tell. But for us baby boomers committed to aging well, it offered some game-changing insights into who we are and how we are seen. As members of a high-risk cohort simply by virtue of the dates on our drivers' licenses, elders were suddenly fragile, in need of extra protection, like an endangered species. Pharmacies scheduled special hours for seniors only. Our grandchildren couldn't even come over to play, much less give us a hug. Kind, friendly, caring neighbors added our shopping lists to theirs and dropped off packages at our doors to shield us from the contagion. Although we appreciated their wonderful generosity of spirit, we found it hard to shake the feeling of confinement.

Some of us would prefer to consider ourselves not all that different from the thirty-five-year-old jogger on the exercise path, or the buff, suntanned blonde rocking it in the Zumba class. This extra protection made us uncomfortable, having to confront the reality that we were different. We were grateful for every day that we weren't coughing, that we could still taste and smell, and that our names weren't listed in the obituaries that tragically included some of our dear friends or acquaintances of long ago.

Many of us were (and are) still working, or deeply involved in community affairs. Though we may have eased up on the urgency and the pressures that had characterized Acts One and Two of our lives, the last thing we had in mind was to be granted our first taste of involuntary retirement. The wind was knocked out of our sails. Sheltering at home didn't have quite the same significance for us as for the younger set; would we ever return to the workplace, or even to the supermarket? It took some effort not to feel just a little bit patronized by those well-intentioned phone calls, checking in with us to make sure we were OK.

We have spoken with many people whose freedom of movement, whether to socialize or to report to a workplace, was curtailed by the pandemic. We've seen a wide range of responses, and we're most impressed with those who have worked through the inevitable anxieties to see such challenging times as a unique opportunity to reclaim and cultivate the power of individual choice. It calls to mind Viktor Frankl's celebration of the inalienable ability every human has to choose a constructive, confident attitude. As we mentioned back in chapter 7, Frankl wrote of the innate liberty we can all access within ourselves to find meaning in any given set of circumstances. One such result we've seen is that as seniors who are more susceptible than younger people, our very presence can inspire those around us, and the rest of the world, to be not only more careful, but more caring. Despite the fear and the unpredictability of these moments, they can be viewed as a microcosm of life under pressure. As our friend Clay says, "The way you do one thing is the way you'll do everything."

We recently heard the story of a certain food distributor who, despite having a beautiful family and a lucrative income, always saw the dark side. His constant negativity and cursing were oppressive to all who knew him. Of all the tasks his business demanded of him, the one he hated most was loading his gourmet yogurts and cheeses into the refrigerator car of a train. He usually assigned this detail to one of his workers, but on one occasion, with no one else around, he had to do it himself. After loading case after case into the refrigerated car, he accidentally pulled the door closed from the inside. There was no way out. He banged on the door, to no avail. The train took off on a thirty-hour journey with him trapped inside. Overcome with the vision of slowly freezing to death, he collapsed to the floor of the car. When the train pulled into the station in San Francisco, workers opened the door and found him unconscious, huddled in the corner. They called an ambulance and he was taken to the ER, with all the signs of severe hypothermia. Strangely, however, there was one thing wrong with this picture. The switch to turn on the refrigerator was discovered in the off position. The refrigerator car was warm, and he survived. His condition had been entirely a product of his attitude, his fear, his fatalistic state of mind.

"Resiliency in Difficult Times" was the topic of a webinar in which we participated not long ago with Tal Ben Shahar, founder of the Harvard School of Positive Psychology. It seemed right up our alley, and we were familiar with Dr. Shahar, who had been kind enough to endorse our work. Pretty much everyone in the helping professions, he said, is familiar with PTSD—post-traumatic stress disorder. Trauma, whether physical or psychological, leaves scars. Traumas might include illness, divorce, accidents, unhappy moves, stress in the workplace, financial loss, difficult children—the battles are many, and the wounds can be devastating. But few people are aware of a scenario that has begun to replace PTSD. It's a concept called PTG, and it stands for *post-traumatic growth*.

Stress is not inherently harmful. Perhaps the best example of that is what happens to our bodies when we go to the gym. We lift weights or perform other exercise regimens that put our bodies under tremendous stress. Then we rest for a day, and we're in better shape than we were before the stress of the workout. The key to gaining the post-traumatic benefit of *growth*, PTG, rather than sustaining injury due to stress, is recovery time: resting appropriately between periods of intense exertion.

Similarly, we can experience extremely stressful situations and thrive, with the proper self-care that provides us recovery time. Whether it is meditation, prayer, aerobic exercise, speaking with a beloved friend, watching a sitcom, or walking along the shore, we can harvest the fruits of stress and heal ourselves to become stronger than we were before.

Many millennials have told us they were at the end of their ropes during the quarantine. Numerous contemporaries, however, told us that it had been the best time of their lives—except for the guilt pangs: what right did they have to be so happy while others were struggling? As seniors, we were the most physically vulnerable segment of the population. Some of us suffered the heart-wrenching loss of loved ones. While the future was shaky and our incomes diminished, it seemed that the quality of some of our closest relationships deepened, even at a distance. Zoom meetings, distance learning, and online interaction with children, grandchildren, and good friends in isolation became our daily rewards. There was extra time for creative projects, for reading and Internet research. Some boomers started new business enterprises and developed a portable career, something they'd been dreaming of for years but had never found the time. Others discovered new hobbies, like backyard gardening or bird watching, or began to journal, eat more naturally, and exercise regularly for the first time in their lives. Some husbands and wives enjoyed a depth of intimacy they had forgotten was possible.

In the midst of pain there was (and there always is) a positive side. During the pandemic, individuals felt as if they were falling apart, but communities seemed to pull together. Neighborhood heroes emerged with various manifestations of helping hands. People waited on socially distanced lines to donate plasma to total strangers. Time once spent walking up and down the aisles of supermarkets and malls was freed up for watercolors, or poetry, or picking up a dust-gathering guitar.

We found out in ways that had never before occurred to us that no one is ever stuck, however confined—or even imprisoned—one might feel. There are as many ways to come unstuck and make life meaningful in the face of chaos as there are hours in the day.

Life is filled with difficult times, and aging well is about living through them, learning from them, and growing stronger and smarter than ever. One choice at a time.

Because the way you do one thing is the way you'll do everything.

Epilogue

Living Your Legacy

The goal isn't to live forever;
the goal is to create something that will.
—CHUCK PALAHNIUK, AUTHOR OF *FIGHT CLUB*

Some people make an indelible impression even when we encounter them only fleetingly. We became acquainted with Robert in 1986, while Simcha was directing a summer fellowship program held at a mountain retreat in upstate New York. Robert was a graduate student at one of America's more prestigious universities, in his mid-twenties, bright, introspective, and inquisitive. What stood out about him was his daily habit of opening *The New York Times* first thing in the morning, not to the sports pages, the book review, the crossword puzzle, or the arts and leisure section, but to the obituaries.

His pensive demeanor offered no clue as to whether this was a morbid fascination or perhaps some sort of sociological interest. We never discussed it. He was just very young to have acquired such an obsession. It seemed almost silly at the time; we were all still young enough to feel more or less invincible.

With our advancing decades, however, every time the idea of death rears its elephant-in-the-room head, it becomes a little less silly. Whenever our sense of mortality sneaks up on us, we recall the image of Robert poring over the obituary page. It's practically impossible not to project oneself into that scenario. At one time or another, doesn't everyone wonder, "What will they write about me when I'm gone?"

The more serious question, however, is, "What is the lasting value of the legacy I will leave?"

Still more intensely personal is the primordial mystery of the afterlife, which is inextricably bound up with our spiritual beliefs: "Where will I be, and who will I be, or will I exist at all? Is there or is there not another kind of life after this life?"

Afterlife scenarios run the gamut from utter denial of the existence of a soul or a spiritual realm to full-blown depictions of heavenly hierarchies. Former skeptics have returned from near-death experiences convinced that they've seen some version of "the light" at the end of whatever tunnel has captured their imagination. Religions have their various theological constructs. Our own tradition is replete with mystical lore that describes, on good authority, the soul's journey through transcendent worlds within worlds. None, however, can define with certainty the true nature of existence in the world to come. Until we get there, even for the faithful, so many questions remain.

We have no intention of proposing definitive answers here. That's probably not a job for any one book, certainly not ours. But we would like to offer a way of taming that wild elephant in the room in a way that renders such meta-physical questions almost moot. Because what matters to us in the here and now is precisely that: what we do *here* and what we can accomplish *right now*.

Whatever our legacies may be, they are the sum total of the ways we conduct ourselves through all the moments of our lifetimes. Act Three may make us a little more nervous about this fact, as we imagine ourselves edging closer to the finish line. But we are more powerful now than we have ever been. Having striven all our lives to be *getting better all the time*, we've gained momentum, experience, and (we daresay) even a smattering of wisdom.

Glancing back through our book, we can see how it culminates here. In Part One, we created a new mission statement for the Third Act, reinventing ourselves, clarifying or redefining our roles and goals. In Part Two, we reconstructed character from the inside out, aligning speech and deeds with heart, mind, and soul; and in Part Three, we put all the ideas to work with methods than can enrich our relationships, our lives, and the lives of others. The elements of a meaningful legacy are now in place. All our thoughts, conversations, and actions represent the growth we've gone through, the milestones we've met, even the errors we've rectified. (*Especially* the errors we've rectified!)

We may or may not have succeeded in realizing every one of our dreams. Have you published your memoirs, painted your masterpiece, or amassed enormous material abundance to pass on to the next generations? Great! If not, also great! Because you're still here, and this glorious moment is at your command. As long as you are present in the moment and unencumbered by the hobgoblins of time, you have all the time in the world. Remembering that, you can express with every gesture who you truly are more wholly and effectively than ever before.

That's where the real legacy becomes evident: in the quality of our lives. If the wheel of fortune has granted us kids and grandkids to keep our surroundings delightfully chaotic, we are not only their genetic forebears—we are their loving role models. We can continue to bestow upon them far more than just our DNA and our probate-protected portfolios. A wry smile in the face of adversity, a calm and trusting response to a stressful situation, an act of kindness toward some stranger who may not deserve it but needs it, could well be the most useful gifts your children or grandchildren will ever receive.

If the younger people around us are not our flesh and blood, we are nonetheless their mentors, their elders, their teachers. We are professors emeritus with advanced degrees from the school of hard knocks. To the extent that we care for them as our students and model for them the worthwhile things we've learned, they are our children as well, and no less our heirs.

Science has long known that tiny causes can have huge effects. In higher mathematics this concept is known as an aspect of chaos theory; in weather prediction and popular culture it's called the *butterfly effect*: when a butterfly flaps its wings in Timbuktu, it can trigger a tornado in Texas. Meteorologists talk about this phenomenon in terms of shifts in the prevailing winds and long, elaborate chains of cause and effect, but in truth it's not just about moving molecules around. It's more subtle than that. It may even happen instantaneously.

The butterfly effect spills over into quantum mechanics, in which a local change can be linked simultaneously to a corresponding change across the globe, or on the other side of the universe. Einstein called it (rather skeptically at the time) *spooky action at a distance.*

This is a principle we would do well to take to heart. One small, seemingly insignificant movement—the wrinkling of the skin, say, in the corner of a smiling eye—can bring joy to the world. Imagine what we can accomplish with big, wide grins; with the sort of kind words, deep teachings, pats on the back, and generous deeds that can put nonstop smiles on sour faces and change temporary darkness into everlasting light.

Go for it. Live your legacy. Be the cause, and the effect will last lifetimes. You don't need to move mountains or believe in eternal life. All it takes is to consider the limitless power of this infinitesimal moment in time and to be genuinely present with the people you love. Your love of life will stir their hearts; your sense of wonder will inspire them with awe. You will live forever in them, and in those they love in turn. *Carpe diem*: seize the day. Age well now, and now, and now. Live the long game. Squeeze the living daylights out of every opportunity that comes your way to keep on being as outrageously awesome as you can be.

And then some.

❧ Appendix ❧

Happier than Ever
Seven Habits That Might Just Make Your Day

These seven suggestions appear in various forms throughout the book—some in great detail, others leaving much more to say. Since our first printing, we've had numerous speaking engagements, and people who've enjoyed the book keep asking for a quick guide, a readily digestible summary of ways to Age Well Now. So here you go:

1. Mindfulness

It's a buzzword these days, and rightfully so. Never before has a generation been so not-present-in-the-moment as ours. Can we stop worrying that we are already late for something that hasn't happened yet?

When we release the baggage of the past and the anxiety that clouds the future, the *now* becomes alive and colorful. In *flow*, we are fully immersed in what we're doing; consciously aware and productive, nonstop; eyes open, alert, and grounded.

This three-breath meditation is a great first step for getting there.

With your first breath, inhale deeply; and as you inhale, feel the energy flow all the way to your feet on the ground, to your bottom on the chair where you sit. Then as you exhale, let go of any and all regrets. The past is the past, and you've done the best you could.

With the next breath, inhale deeply again; be aware of your lungs and all your organs, and how they faithfully nourish you from within. As you exhale, let go of any worries about the future—even tomorrow, even ten minutes from now. What is about to happen is an open book. Why let the unknowable sap your energy, your focus, your joy?

With the third breath, inhale deeply, and feel your connection to all the good you have shared with the world, to the beautiful person you are inside, and your positive, powerful potential. As you exhale come fully present into the *now*, with gratitude, focus, clarity, and calm.

Claim your flow!

2. Connection

Harvard's eighty-year Study of Adult Development revealed that the primary indicator for happiness and longevity is the quality of our *relationships*. Healthy bonds with family and friends bode well for a positive future, far more than financial status, professional accomplishments, and even self-care.

Make time for family. Schedule it in your calendar and to-do list. Make it as nonnegotiable as your next dental appointment. A family chat on WhatsApp is great, but it won't take the place of in-the-flesh connection, hugs, dinners, and walks in the park.

Reach out to old friends.

Take an active role in your local community.

Practice forgiveness, and don't take things personally.

Connect to your Source/Creator on a daily basis, through prayer or meditation. Catch a wave that's much bigger than you.

3. Gratitude

People who practice gratitude regularly experience more positive emotions, feel more alive, sleep better, express more compassion and kindness, and even have stronger immune systems. University of California psychologist Robert Emmons tells us that gratitude actually rewires the brain.

Keep a gratitude notebook. Each day, write down three things you're grateful for, record one pleasant moment, and acknowledge one small personal victory. ("I only had two pieces of seven-layer cake when I really wanted three!")

Say thank you to as many people as you can, wherever you are.

4. Self-Discipline

Every act of self-control is an act of self-respect. Try to eat only when sitting down. Be careful not to interrupt others when they're speaking. Don't complain or gossip between 5:00 and 7:00 p.m. Try to stay off your phone until 9:30 a.m.—even one day a week for starters.

Be sure to write these personal victories in your gratitude notebook.

5. Positive Thinking and Speaking

Try to refine your expressions, and your thoughts will follow. Avoid the drama. Things look brighter when we are not alarmists or awfulizers: your subconscious mind responds to such messages as though they were real.

Is your headache *really* "killing you"? Is it true that you "*can't stand* your child? Is your significant other literally a "pain in the butt"?

"Always" and "never" are temperamental words, are seldom accurate, and tend to eclipse the good that others have done. ("You *never* help me." "You're *always* late.")

6. Self-Care

When you take the time for a foot massage, a meaningful journal entry, a hot shower, a five-minute meditation, or a restorative yoga class, you give yourself the message that you're worth it. And you really are.

Set aside time every day for yourself, even if it's only a ten-minute walk. Make yourself a power drink every morning. And be sure to make your bed.

Don't blame anyone else for your unhappiness or lackluster life. Be proactive, and let it shine. Make a list of things you'd love to do; treat yourself to one each week.

7. Routine

Strange as it may seem, a well-established routine allows us to be more spontaneous. There is a certain joy and sense of stability in seeing the patterns in our day and week. Many diets emphasize the importance of eating at the same time everyday. Waking and sleeping on schedule are also excellent aids for lowering stress. When you have a clear idea of what to expect each day, you're able to plan those lovely excursions and reunions with family and friends—because you can see the space in your schedule rather than feeling overwhelmed or vaguely committed to something, but you're not sure what.

Order brings peace to the soul.

Notes

Chapter 1

1. Jane Fonda, *Life's Third Act*, TED Talk, December 2011: https://www.ted.com/talks/jane_fonda_life_s_third_act.

2. Gary Small, MD, *Two Weeks to a Younger Brain* (West Palm Beach, Fla.: Humanix Books, 2015).

3. Lewis Carroll, *Alice's Adventures in Wonderland and Through the Looking Glass* (New York: Bantam Dell, 1981 [1865]).

4. Edgar Rice Burroughs, *Tarzan of the Apes* (London: Dalton House, 2015).

Chapter 2

5. Janet Bray Attwood and Chris Attwood, *The Passion Test* (Fairfield, Iowa: First World Publishing, 2006).

6. Stephen R. Covey, *Focus: Achieving Your Highest Priorities.* Audio workshop: FranklinCovey, 2004.

7. Babylonian Talmud, *Ethics of the Fathers* 1:14.

Chapter 3

8. Rabbi Abraham Ben Meir Ibn Ezra (1089–1167). Popularized in the nineteenth century as a song. Born in Spain, Ibn Ezra was one of the most distinguished Jewish poets and philosophers of the Middle Ages.

9. "Gum Disease and the Connection to Heart Disease," Harvard Medical School Health Publications (website), April 2018: www.health.harvard.edu/press_releases/heart-disease-oral-health.

10. Tal Ben Shahar, *Happier* (New York: McGraw Hill, 2007).

11. Tony Schwartz, *The Power of Full Engagement* (New York: Simon and Schuster, 2005).

12. Robert Emmons and Michael McCullough, *The Psychology of Gratitude* (London: Oxford University Press, 2004).

Chapter 4

13. Mihaly Csikszentmihalyi, *Flow* (New York: Harper and Row, 1990).

Chapter 5

14. Jon Kabat Zinn, *Mindfulness for Beginners* (Boulder, Colo.: Sounds True, 2012).

15. Herbert Benson, MD, and Miriam Z. Klipper, *The Relaxation Response* (New York: Harper Collins, 2000).

Chapter 6

16. Bob Smith, MD, and Bill Wilson, *The Big Book of Alcoholics Anonymous* (New York: Lark, 2013 [1939]).

17. Daniel Goleman, PhD, *Emotional Intelligence: Why It Can Matter More Than IQ* (New York: Bantam, 1995).

18. W. Mischel, E.B. Ebbesen, and A.R. Zeiss, "Cognitive and Attentional Mechanisms in Delay of Gratification," *Journal of Personality and Social Psychology* 21, no. 2 (Feb. 1972): 204-218.

19. Shawn Achor, *The Happy Secret to Better Work*. TED Talk, Sept. 2011: https://www.ted.com/talks/shawn_achor_the_happy_secret_to_better_work?language=en.

20. Stephen R. Covey, *The Seven Habits of Highly Effective People* (New York: Simon and Schuster, 1990), 235–60.

Chapter 7

21. Daniel T. Gilbert and Mathew A. Killingsworth, "A Wandering Mind Is an Unhappy Mind," *Science* 330, no. 6006 (Nov. 12, 2010): 932: DOI: 10.1126/science.1192439.

22. Larry Kim, "Multitasking Is Killing Your Brain," *Observer*, Feb. 2, 2016: http://observer.com/2016/02/multitasking-is-killing-your-brain/.

23. Fred Luskin, *Forgive for Good: A Proven Prescription for Health and Happiness* (New York: Harper Collins, 2002).

24. Viktor Frankl, *Man's Search for Meaning* (Boston: Beacon Press, 2006).

25. Colin Tipping, *Radical Forgiveness* (Boulder, Colo.: Sounds True, 2009).

26. Miriam Adahan, *Awareness: The Key to Acceptance, Forgiveness, and Growth* (New York: Feldheim, 1994).

Chapter 8

27. Bill Newcott, "The Paradox of Prayer," *AARP Magazine*, February-March, 2015, 48-52, 86.

28. Frank Newport, "Most Americans Believe in God," Gallup (website), June 29, 2016: http://www.gallup.com/poll/193271/americans-believe-god.aspx.

Chapter 9

29. Gary Chapman, *The Five Love Languages* (Chicago: Northfield, 2015).

30. Covey, *Seven Habits*, 237.

Chapter 10

31. Kara Mayer Robinson, "Ten Surprising Health Benefits of Sex," WebMD Archives (website), accessed Jan. 29, 2021: http://www.webmd.com/sex-relationships/guide/sex-and-health#1.

32. Tiffany Field, PhD, *Touch* (Boston: MIT Press, 2001).

Chapter 11

33. Covey, *Seven Habits*, 188ff.

Chapter 12

34. "Living Wills and Advance Directives for Health Decisions," Mayo Clinic Consumer Health (website), accessed Jan. 29, 2021: http://www.mayoclinic.org/healthy-lifestyle/consumer-health/in-depth/living-wills/art-20046303.

Chapter 13

35. David Hamilton, *Why Kindness Is Good for You* (Carlsbad, Calif.: Hay House, 2010).

36. Julia Cameron, *The Artist's Way* (New York: Penguin Putnam, 2002).

Chapter 14

37. Nikolaos Scarmeas, MD, Nicole Schupf, PhD, et al., "Physical Activity, Diet, and Alzheimer Disease" *JAMA*, Aug. 12, 2009: DOI:10.1001/jama.2009.1144.

38. Ephrat Livni, "The Japanese Practice of Forest Bathing Is Scientifically Proven to Improve Your Health," Quartz (website), Oct. 12, 2016: https://qz.com/804022/health-benefits-japanese-forest-bathing.

39. Max Hirshkowitz, PhD, Kaitlyn Whiton, MHS, et al., "National Sleep Foundation's Sleep Time Recommendations," *Sleep Health* 1, no. 1 (March 2015): 40–43: http://dx.doi.org/10.1016/j.sleh.2014.12.010.

Acknowledgments

We owe a debt of gratitude to many benevolent souls, without whom this book may not have seen the light of day. Among them:

Meir Michel Abehsera, for whom magic, humor, and poetry were daily fare; who taught that to be truly alive is to follow your dream; and who showed us that it's OK to take a long time to write a book.

Bruce and Rivka, Eli and Chana, and Avi and Baila, for providing perfect places for our writing retreats, where inertia could surrender to momentum.

Bev Buncher, who believed in us from the start and guided us toward the right connections.

John Eggen and Christy Tryhus, who coached us, and coached us some more, and helped us gain traction in our slip-slidey lives.

Hal Strauss, who astutely edited our manuscript, then told us it's a good book.

The elderly gentleman jogging every morning along the canal, whose twinkly eye reminds us how all the scary scuttlebutt about aging can't possibly be real.

Mr. Canell, Simcha's eleventh-grade English teacher, who between tirades against the slovenly decadence of bourgeois youth exclaimed with surprise, "You write English!"

The countless other professors, prophets, revolutionaries, mentors, healers, teachers, coaches, and provocateurs who have disrupted our lives—to our betterment as well as that of humanity; and the equally innumerable students, patients, clients, campers, mentees, readers, customers, and kids, who ask the questions and pose the problems that prod us to grow, and keep us in flow.

Rabbi Menachem Mendel Schneerson, who imbued in us an understanding of how much good a single individual can accomplish when connected above, and who modeled the dedication it takes to get it done.

The Creator of the Universe, Who continuously brings this glorious reality into existence and grants us life, that we may play out all three acts in vibrant color, and in the flesh.

About the Authors

Through her career as a beloved teacher, educational consultant, outreach director, and principal of one of America's largest private day schools, Frumma Rosenberg-Gottlieb has touched and transformed thousands of lives. She now devotes her time to coaching, speaking, and writing, primarily in the realms of personal growth, healthy relationships, and emotional intelligence. Quoted as an expert on mindfulness in *Time* magazine and by Arianna Huffington in her book *Thrive*, Frumma has also appeared on *The Oprah Winfrey Show* and is featured in the *New York Times* best seller *Small Miracles*.

Simcha Gottlieb, an acupuncture physician and doctor of Oriental medicine, sees health and well-being from the integrated, whole-systems perspective of body, mind, and soul. With a long prior career to his credit as a pioneering writer, producer, and filmmaker, today Simcha is a respected wellness coach, teacher of meditation, spiritual mentor, and demystifier of mysticism. Several of his works on the clinical implications of consciousness and wholesome lifestyle have been published internationally.

Together Frumma and Simcha have traveled to far corners of the planet, sharing their insights on joy, creativity, and a life well lived. Between them they have raised thirteen wonderful adult children and more than twice that number of grandchildren (but who's counting?).

To contact Simcha and Frumma Gottlieb for speaking engagements, workshops, retreats, and individual coaching, visit their website at www.age-well-now.com.

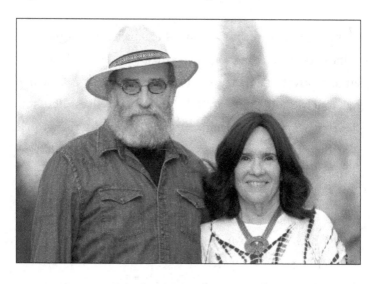

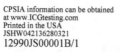

CPSIA information can be obtained
at www.ICGtesting.com
Printed in the USA
JSHW042136280321
12990JS00001B/1